For every carer, part of an undervalued workforce, who struggles to survive the daily grind of caring for a loved one, often with little acknowledgement and less thanks.

Endurance: It is the spirit which can bear things, not simply with resignation but with blazing hope. It is the quality which keeps a man on his feet with his face to the wind. It is the virtue which can transmute the hardest trial into glory because beyond the pain it sees the goal.

Come be My Follower
Anonymous

Acknowledgements

I would like to thank Henry Butterfield who guided me away from schoolgirl English and assured me that I had a story to tell.

Thanks also to Laura Kamel who took the time to tidy up my atrocious spelling and grammar.

A huge thank you to my wonderful son, who has accepted my need to write this book.

And finally, thanks to John Gayton for allowing me to use his photograph of a Hocking's ice cream van in Bideford for the cover.

Jill Stoking

PART 1

Chapter One

'Bob, where's my handbag? I can't find it. I must have left it in Sainsbury's.'

My mother's voice quivers with panic. I've only been here for three days, but I'm irritated by her childish tone and the "hunt the handbag" ritual is wearing thin.

Dad, slumped in his armchair, watches cricket on the TV. People who really know my father would describe him as possessing a short fuse. I should know, I'd received the full force of the blast enough times. The telltale sign was always his tongue, which had a life of its own. When he was in contemplative mood, it would snake out of the corner of his mouth and curl over the top lip into his moustache. However, seconds before an explosion, the tongue would protrude between his taut lips only to be clamped by his teeth to form a blood engorged slug. It was a useful warning signal for the recipient of wrath, usually me. It's just that I'd never learnt how to defuse him.

Dad doesn't respond as I would have predicted. This must be the sixth time today that Mum has mislaid her handbag. He seems quite calm, no tongue, no raised voice and no foul language.

'I don't expect it's far away, Poppet.'

His voice is modulated to placate, it almost caresses. I'm unnerved by his laid-back response. I assume the pose of co-conspirator, as my mother continues to wander from room to room, searching.

'Doesn't this constant handbag fixation drive you nuts?'

'I suppose I've got used to it.' He shrugs.

'It's okay I've found it!' A triumphant cry. Then Mum's sheepish face peeps round the door of the lounge.

'There you are, Poppet,' says Dad. 'I told you it would turn up.'

***

That was in 1988 and probably the first inkling that my mother, Joan, was developing Alzheimer's disease. For me, it wasn't a conscious realisation. She'd always been a wife who was eager to please her husband, one of the "old school". I can remember, when I was a child, my mother would spend an hour before the dressing table mirror transforming herself into a domestic goddess from "The Good Wife Guide". Dress on, powder and lipstick applied, pristine frilly apron tied around her tiny waist, ready for my father to arrive home from the office. She would always have his dinner prepared and on the table by the time he'd changed out of his city suit into his scruffy casual gear. No dinners on trays in our house.

Mum seemed nervous of having an opinion that wasn't shared by my father. *Being a dizzy dame when you were in your twenties might have been attractive,* I thought, *but the dumb blonde act now that you're in your sixties just makes you look senile.*

I never thought it might have been the start of just that. The pieces only fell into place with hindsight. It's a relatively useless thing, hindsight.

***

My parents were still living in a mock Tudor semi in New Malden, South West London. Dad had bought the house before World War II and lived there with his first wife. Mum successfully ousted wife number one after a wartime affair leaked into peacetime. She wasn't prepared to let her sergeant major lover escape back into domestic oblivion.

I'd moved to Devon in the mid-seventies and a decade later my brother, Bob, and his family, had moved from Sutton, technically still in Surrey, to Devon and now lived a few miles away from me.

Bob had begun his life in the West Country, as the landlord of a village pub. He'd been in partnership with an old school friend, but had been forced to sell up when his business partner had wanted out. Bob still lived in the same village with his wife, Marie, and their two daughters. I'd moved from the rural dream to the outskirts of Bideford and had an ailing marriage, one son and a succession of part-time jobs that fitted around motherhood.

Our plan had been that Mum and Dad would move down to the West Country to be near us. Dad refused to budge.

'I'm not uprooting myself just to salve your conscience.'

That statement had been thrown in my face when I broached the subject of moving. He wouldn't have said that to Bob, their relationship was very close. After Dad's death, we found evidence that he'd begun to contemplate a move to be closer to the support of his children. By then, he must have found it difficult to cope, though he'd hidden it extremely well.

***

When I moved to Devon, my parents used to come for a holiday two or three times a year and stayed with me. For the last few years, they'd chosen to stay with my brother. I would go up to visit them, with my son Jake, a couple of times during the year, but those visits had become increasingly tense.

That homecoming in 1988 had begun badly. My mother had fallen up the steps at Paddington Station. She was beginning to fall over quite a bit by this time, but there was always a plausible reason why she appeared to trip over fresh air. On this particular occasion, Mum claimed she'd been pushed by somebody trying to get past her. There were no witnesses, it appeared to have been a push and run job.

I stepped off the train, with a tired and hungry young son, to be confronted by Mum, being very brave. Dad looked sick, pathetic and irritated all at the same time, with the aura of expectation that I'd perform my capable daughter act and sort it.

Mum had sustained a deep gash down the line of her shinbone which needed hospital attention. I found a policeman, who, having glanced at her leg, gave us a police escort to St Thomas' Hospital, where we spent the next three hours waiting for my mother's leg to be treated with steri-strips. That was followed by the inevitable daily visits to the health centre to have the dressing changed. Strangely, she never felt any pain with it and the wound healed well.

During a previous visit that same year, Mum had managed to drop a casserole dish full of sweet and sour pork while lifting it out of the oven. The contents had splattered over her feet and legs. My mother had always been capable in a crisis, it shouldn't have needed me to give her first aid advice, but as she stood there, not making a move to do anything constructive, I felt obliged to issue instructions.

'Go and sit on the edge of the bath and put your feet in cold water while I clear this mess up.'

It's surprising how far a dish of stew will travel and it took a while to retrieve bits of pork from under the fridge and cooker. My father appeared at the kitchen door some twenty minutes later.

'Is it okay if she takes her feet out of the bath now? They've gone blue with the cold.'

My son Jake and I had developed survival tactics for these visits. If I started to get too irritated with my mother, we had a code word that Jake would aim in my direction, in an attempt to tell me to stop the rant. In this instance he gave up, I was past listening.

For me these visits were proving to be almost as stressful as being at home with a husband who'd stopped having anything to do with me on virtually any level, years ago. We just happened to live, uneasily, within the same house.

***

Later that year Dad had to go into hospital for an operation to reduce an enlarged prostate. This was a problem that had become more than a mild inconvenience and required the carrying of a suitable receptacle in the car at all times to pee into when he got caught short, which was often. Mum coped quite well. I went up and stayed for a while until Dad came out of hospital, but was unable to visit again when, a week later, he had to be readmitted because he was passing blood. She managed on her own, and I was mildly surprised.

In 1992, a few months before his eightieth birthday, Dad made the announcement that he couldn't travel to Devon anymore to see his family, it was too much for him. If his children wanted to see him, we'd have to go to New Malden.   They did come to Devon once more, after that proclamation, Christmas 1993, mainly at my mother's instigation, I think. She'd always been partial to a medical drama, and I'd recently had a biopsy on my breast. I was still waiting to hear if it was benign or sinister. I have a photograph of Dad, sitting in my brother's lounge, more than half-cut.

That Christmas was the last time I saw him.

***

Aged eighty-one, Dad was still playing golf twice a week with a golfing partner of many years acquaintance. They never socialised at any other time and our families had never met. Geoff had spoken to my mother on the phone if he rang to cancel a game, which rarely happened. Geoff, by all accounts, was a competent and controlled golfer. My father was an erratic, bad-tempered and expletive-spouting opponent. After their game, they would adjourn to the clubhouse for liquid refreshment, a cup of coffee for Geoff and a pint of bitter for Dad, before going their separate ways.

Under the circumstances, I felt genuine sympathy for Geoff when Dad dropped dead on the way back to the clubhouse after a round of eighteen holes. Dead before he hit the ground. 11th January, 1994.

Geoff had the unenviable task of telling my mother, a woman he didn't know, that her husband wasn't coming home. Ever. Like the true gentleman I'd always pictured him to be, he escorted Mum to the hospital. Understandably, she wanted to go there immediately. The hospital staff hadn't had time to prepare Dad's body for viewing, which compounded her distress.

'I couldn't believe he was dead, I wasn't going to believe it unless I saw him for myself, but they'd taken his teeth out,' she said.

Geoff came to the funeral and that was that. With his golfing partner gone, there was no reason to remain in contact.

My brother received the call about my father's death from Mum's next door neighbours, a young couple whose two small children were regular recipients of my mother's child minding skills. Bob immediately came round to tell me. He was devastated, and I was upset by his grief, though quite numb to the cause of it. I didn't feel very much at all and still don't to this day. My father and I had an uneasy relationship, and my memories of Dad aren't totally shared by my brother. But then, Bob says he can't remember many details at all from his childhood.

Bob had been a delicate child. Bronchial pneumonia at nine months old, tonsils out in early childhood and then a condition called purpura, which meant that you only had to look at him and he appeared to erupt in bruises. This type of purpura required a lengthy hospital stay in Queen Mary's Hospital for Children in Carshalton. More significantly, he received gifts with every visit, a ritual to which I was always an envious onlooker.

Once returned to the loving arms of his parents, the usual sparring and physical rivalry between siblings was forbidden. Bob was treated as a delicate child and placed off limits to his only sister, who'd hated him since birth and daily plotted ways to rid herself of this alien interloper. It also rendered him untouchable to a father who had a nasty temper. It seemed to me that I got double rations of that temper.

On the day Dad died, Bob and I travelled up from Devon to be with Mum. During the days leading up to the funeral, both of us came to the conclusion that she was far from 'with it'. Not as tearful as we'd expected, but vacant and removed from the situation. Shell-shocked was the expression that came to mind. We attributed it to grief, thinking that the tears would inevitably come later, when the reality of Dad's death penetrated her fragile veneer.

My father's funeral was like a scene from a soap opera. Both Dad and Bob were professed atheists, Mum had never expressed the slightest inclination toward any religion, Christian or otherwise and I was, and still am, one of Jehovah's Witnesses. Either a civil or a humanist funeral was a contender that appeared to appease the sensibilities of the majority. We hadn't taken into account a mother who, it seemed, suddenly got God. She decided on a Church of England service, and nothing was going to dissuade her.

Bob contacted the undertakers who arranged for the duty vicar to visit. He was a pleasant man who was no doubt accustomed to people fostering a religious faith following bereavement, a touchstone in times of distress and uncertainty. Mum, now stuck in a situation she'd no idea how to handle, escaped into the grieving widow role and remained damp-eyed and mute throughout the entire visit.

The poor guy, flummoxed and floundering, turned to my brother and asked in his cut glass voice, 'Did your father believe in the resurrection?'

Bob explained that he and his father were atheists and his sister was one of Jehovah's Witnesses, so he'd no idea why our mother was insisting on a service that her husband would have hated. I personally thought that this little speech was delivered with more relish than was strictly necessary. To give the vicar his due, he appeared sympathetic and agreed to keep the doctrine to a minimum, apart from the bits he was obliged to include. He was as good as his word.

At the crematorium, I remained dry-eyed and detached throughout the entire service. Mum, standing stoically by my side, seemed similarly removed from the proceedings. Bob, however, admitted that he was digging his fingernails into his leg to prevent himself from breaking down. Strange, how two children from the same family can feel so differently towards a parent. The one fact we did both agree on, was that Mum wasn't going to cope well with life without her husband.

Food and drink had been prepared for the few we anticipated would come back to the family home after the funeral. We'd underestimated the number of relatives and friends, some not seen for years, who turned up. Neither did we foresee the amount of alcohol friends and relatives were able to consume because it was free.

One second cousin, a lad of eighteen or so, who I'd met about three times and Bob didn't remember at all, binged on brandy. It was an attempt to numb the pain of his own personal bereavement, the termination of his first love affair. He went on a drunken rampage through the quiet suburban streets. He managed to demolish a neighbour's garden wall and render damage to a parked vehicle before Bob and Jim, who was a cousin and retired policeman, caught up with him and gave him a severe talking to. Bob had the unenviable task of visiting the recipients of the vandalism, offering payment and words of appeasement and regret. We never did receive an apology.

Chapter Two

My father's Christian names were Charles Robert, but he was always known as Bob and my brother, whose name was Robert Charles, went by the name of Robert, until the death of his father. From the moment Dad died, everyone began calling my brother by the derivative form of his name — Bob. Like an inheritance, accepted without comment by anyone, as if it was a birthright.

Bob cleared as much of the mountain of paperwork as he could during the week of the funeral. It became apparent that Dad had hoarded bills, bank statements and correspondence going back over a decade. It was going to be a mammoth task to sort through and reorganise his system into something workable for Mum to take over. The next shock was my mother's total inability to take over anything. She'd never written a cheque, changed a light bulb or paid a bill and she wasn't in the frame of mind to start, or so it seemed.

Fortunately, Dad had made a will, leaving everything to Mum. Even so, the amount of letters, phone calls and certified copies of the will and death certificate required to put everything into her name, was time-consuming. Even to me it was overwhelming. Bob coped with it all and arranged for utility bills and insurances to be paid by direct debit. He also obtained joint authority over Mum's bank account, so we could, if necessary, withdraw money on her behalf.

Meanwhile, I was attempting, with little success, to teach my mother how to write a cheque, use the lawnmower and help her sort through Dad's personal belongings, some for immediate disposal, others not to be parted with just yet, if at all.

During that week, we discovered the Red Book. Dad had kept a record of every financial transaction since the end of World War II, including money he'd lent to Bob and me. I noticed, with a touch of cynicism, that many of the loans he'd made to my brother had a strike through them with the words "written off".

The one and only loan he'd made to me, for repairing a roof, some seventeen years before, was left with the final ten pounds of the repayments still outstanding. I remembered the event. I was paying Dad back when I got paid, at a rate of ten pounds a month. I was convinced that I'd repaid the whole loan, Dad disputed it. Neither of us was prepared to budge on the issue, so that ten pounds remained in his Red Book as "debt unpaid".

Bob and I drew much closer during that week. I'd always resented him, feeling that he'd been the favourite, but hadn't realised that he felt the same way about me. Talking together, while engrossed in the sorting out process and the reminiscence that inevitably follows the death of a parent, we came to understand that our parents had played us off against each other all our lives.

That came as a shock, but also a healing. For the first time in my forty-three years, I came to recognize that I had a brother who was similar to me in many ways, and I was actually beginning to like him.

***

I thought I'd known the character of my parents, their strengths and weaknesses, likes and dislikes. But moving away from home and out of the area in my early twenties, I'd lost that intimacy, presuming I ever had it. Bob had remained nearby for a lot longer and Dad, post retirement, had even worked for him for a while. We both thought that our parents, although not short of money, weren't exactly flush either. I suppose we were both basing this on the condition of the house and contents.

Dad never bought anything if he could make it. Hence wardrobes were all custom built, by Dad, with timber that would have been more suitable for the construction of an air raid shelter. The dining room furniture was pre-war, but shop bought and had been in situ during the reign of his first wife. The bathroom tiling was the original 1930s. The kitchen had been designed, made and fitted by my father.

The house still had the original separate lounge and dining room, while most of the street had opted for converting the two rooms into one. The lounge was south facing and well lit through bay windows. The dining room faced north and was always dingy and cold. The stereo unit, TV unit and coffee tables were all constructed out of veneered chipboard with screw in black legs. If you unwittingly flopped down on the settee, you were likely to break your spine on the board placed under the cushions to bolster the base of the settee, which had sagged irreversibly. Uncharacteristically, Dad had acquired double glazing quite recently, so perhaps he'd begun to make moves towards joining the twentieth century.

The garden hadn't fared much better. The vegetable patch, an invaluable space during the war when it'd been utilised to supplement a meagre diet, had long since been grassed over. A piece of land had been sold to a neighbour, who'd wanted to build a garage on it, and Dad had acquired a garage too. That was it, on the improvement front. The two pre-war apple trees remained standing, though riddled with disease, and the much-patched garden shed was being held together by ingrown honeysuckle.

It was the same shed that I'd used at a very young age as a pretend horse-drawn caravan. My push-along horse had been hitched to the shed by my skipping rope and numerous tennis balls in the role of sheep were scattered over the sparse lawn. I was, by turn, the gypsy herder and the sheepdog, barking my way over the cracked clay ground to round up the flock. It had also served as somewhere to sleep at night when, as an out of control teenager, I'd return home, in the early hours of the morning, to find myself locked out of the house and the spare key, normally hidden in the shed, removed.

So, it came as something of a surprise, to discover that Mum's assets were very healthy indeed and it made that outstanding debt, entered in the

Red Book, appear to me to be mean minded. When we sat her down and explained that she wouldn't have any money worries, Mum appeared to be genuinely shocked and embarrassed by the amount involved, claiming that she'd no idea that they'd acquired such a large sum.

I have a theory that Dad was stockpiling money with the intention of putting them both into a residential care home if, or when, the time came, rather than be a burden, an inconvenience, or just beholden to his children. I certainly believe that my mother had exhibited signs of dementia, for some eight years or more, prior to Dad's death.

***

My marriage, at the time of my father's death, was beyond salvaging. Although we lived in the same house, Ray hadn't spoken to me for the last seven years. The act of subjecting me to the silent treatment had always been his way of bringing me to heel if, in his view, I'd erred in any way and appeared unrepentant.

The first time this tactic had been used was soon after we began living together. Ray felt, with some justification, that it was inappropriate for the senior administrative officer and the filing clerk (me) to be living together and still working in the same department. He wanted me to change my job. I was in no hurry to leave. He hastened the process by refusing to speak to me. I stuck it out for six weeks, then caved in and applied for a transfer to another department in a different building.

The relationship warmed up and at the end of 1977 we progressed from cohabitation to marriage. By the time I was pregnant with Jake, in 1981, we'd bought a house, but the marriage was in trouble.

I knew he wasn't in love with me, and looking back, I don't believe he ever was. It was the classic tale of a relationship entered into on the rebound in the vain hope that it will make the beneficiary of unrequited love realise what she'd carelessly discarded. His ex-girlfriend obviously hadn't read the script. Penny had forfeited her affair with Ray and left her husband, with whom she still lived, for a much younger man. She enjoyed (or not) living with him for a while before she returned to her husband and bore him three sons.

The week after Ray and I moved in together, I'd received a phone call at work from somebody unknown to me. She felt it was in my best interest to know that Ray was still involved with his ex-girlfriend. Ray hotly denied the allegation, of course.

I honestly thought that Ray would leave me when I told him I was pregnant. I had, as far as possible, mentally prepared myself for that event. He'd always said that he didn't want children, but at thirty-one, my biological clock was ticking loud enough to drown out misgivings. I'd selfishly reasoned that if I was going to lose him anyway, at least I'd have part of him in his child. I was in love with Ray, I couldn't imagine I would ever want to be with anyone else and I didn't want a child with anyone but Ray. I'm sure he wanted to leave, but I hadn't factored in his sense of duty.

Reflecting on it afterwards, his mother would never have forgiven him if he'd abandoned his wife and unborn child, which may have had some bearing on his decision to stay. Ray certainly wasn't happy at the news and I spent three days "in Coventry". As there wasn't going to be a U-turn on this issue, he blotted out the inevitable with a seven month bender and the declaration, to anyone who'd listen, that he wasn't the father. He had the names of two men who he considered were plausible candidates and bandied around one name or the other, depending on which group of bar room cronies he was with at the time. On the surface, I took this gross insult as a joke, because that's how it was presented. He never knew how emotionally bruised he made me feel.

Ray stayed with me during the lengthy labour and birth, which surprised me a bit. Jake was born on 26th November, 1981, a healthy eight and a quarter pounds in old money. The next day, Ray was the first visitor to the maternity unit, and he brought flowers. He was also drunk and went into the wrong ward and presented the wrong mother with the bouquet. I later learnt that the flowers had been given to him by a regular in the pub, where Ray had wet the baby's head.

The marriage slowly slid from bad to worse. Drunken nastiness, emotional abuse and periods of silence were its hallmark. When Jake was a year old, I started studying the Bible with Jehovah's Witnesses. I'd never read the Bible, had no religious inclination, but accepted the study, initially as an academic exercise because my brain felt atrophied. Ray was horrified and declared that he hated me for what I was doing. My brain was being stretched and I wanted to continue and was genuinely baffled by this outpouring of blind prejudice. It was the excuse he needed, the peg to hang our failed marriage on. He could officially blame my involvement with Jehovah's Witnesses and thereby move the responsibility onto my shoulders.

Whenever I hear somebody asserting that Jehovah's Witnesses break up marriages, I have to fight myself to hold back the retort, 'Whatever went on before, behind closed doors, broke up the marriage, not Jehovah's Witnesses.'

The fact is, they do their utmost to give you scriptural counsel to enable you to repair your relationship, but both partners need to want the marriage to work. Ray didn't.

The last time Ray spoke to me conversationally in our domestic environment was March, 1985. The shutters came down for the last time. His physical presence was evident by the atmosphere in the home, which you could almost slice and dice. We lived in the same house, but had separate lives and after the first silent year, separate bedrooms. I grieved for the husband I was still in love with. But I guess Ray would tell a different story.

***

After the funeral, I decided to bring Mum back with me to Bideford to stay with my brother for a couple of weeks. I needed to keep a post-op hospital appointment at Barnstaple, to discover what had been removed from my breast. I never did find out. The registrar bounced in with the good news that it was benign. Having waited for six weeks to hear the results, I wanted details, but he obviously hadn't been briefed about what had actually been removed. His suggestion was a visit to my GP who'd be informed by letter. I felt my tolerance level come to an abrupt halt so, tight lipped, I left.

***

Mum seemed so pathetic and lost. I found it hard to imagine that she was ever going to be reconciled to being on her own.

'It's the grief, she'll need time,' my brother said.

Bob had worked as an insurance agent and he'd seen this before many times when dealing with the newly bereaved. I wanted to believe him, but there was this nagging doubt. I recalled the last few years of weekly telephone conversations with my mother, which had become repeats of the week before. The continuity of the stuff of life had ceased and I'd become quite resentful.

'She doesn't care. She's not interested in my life or what her only grandson is doing.'

Now I wasn't at all sure if that had been the case. The lost handbag issue, my father's uncharacteristic patience with her, his refusal to come to Devon anymore, all began to ring alarm bells. Had Dad begun to find it hard to compensate for her failing faculties?

I was employed as a care assistant at a nursing home and had looked after many elderly people with the late stages of dementia, when they'd exhausted friends and relatives to the point where they could no longer look after their loved one at home. But I had no experience of the symptoms that marked the early phases of this cruel disease. I was about to enter new territory and undertake a journey that would prove to be devastating for Mum.

***

For the next nine months, my life became a complex juggling act that involved part-time work and the struggle to maintain the pretence of normal family life. Now, I had to fit in monthly visits to New Malden, slotted into the midweek period when I wasn't on duty at the nursing home.

My mother struggled to cope. Mail would flop through her door and, to her, it was all equally important and the cause of extreme anxiety. She couldn't distinguish between junk mail and missives to be dealt with and was totally unable to read anything with comprehension. Light bulbs blew and she was unable to learn how to change them. The grass needed to be cut, but my mother couldn't work the lawn mower. A neighbour told me that she'd attempted to push an electric lawn mower around the garden, without the benefit of electricity. He kindly took on that particular task, and he and his wife took Mum shopping to Sainsbury's, once a week.

Not one of my visits went by without my mother throwing a tantrum over something. On one memorable occasion, I'd loaded her car up with junk from the garden shed, in an attempt to reduce the amount of father-induced hoarded things, which might prove useful. The plan was to offload the rubbish at the municipal dump and then do a big shop at the supermarket, but Mum had got it into her head that we were shopping first.

On the A3, she lost it and threw a major wobbly. She began to scream, her mouth stretched wide open, as she pulled at her hair with both fists in an attempt to tear it from her head while she drummed her feet, in a tattoo, on the floor of the car. My instinctive reaction, though I'm not proud of it, was to slap her across the legs while still negotiating an extremely busy road. Mercifully, the hysteria abruptly stopped. The incident left me shocked and appalled, not only because of my act of physical chastisement, but also that my mother had thrown a temper tantrum typical of a two-year-old. I experienced an epiphany. This situation was not going to get better. Time to rethink.

Chapter Three

It's always been the accepted advice that, after bereavement, it's best to shelve plans to relocate for a couple of years. I didn't see the two year breathing space as an option in my mother's case.

Bob and I discussed the problem at length and decided that the only realistic plan was for her to move to Devon, near us. At this point, we still expected that Mum's inability to function would stabilise, if she had more support from her family. The hope was that when she'd come to terms with her loss, and if her anxiety levels could be reduced, then maybe she'd be able to make a life for herself.

Leaving friends behind wasn't an issue. Dad had been an insular person, the few friends they had, drifted away after his death. Mum had been in the same house all her married life, plus some, but had recently disclosed that she disliked the place. Nothing in it was her choice and the house had originally been the marital home of my father and his first wife.

I'd never realised she felt that way, but I was still coming to terms with the knowledge that Dad had been married before. Bob and I only found out a few years prior to his death, when I'd received an anonymous letter, presumably from a relative. This reptile was incensed over a legacy Dad had received from his stepmother's sister, as reward for some administrative assistance. The author of the letter felt that the inherited money should have been shared between Dad's siblings. In an attempt to portray my father as a devious, untrustworthy ne'er do well, the writer decided to illustrate that point by informing me that Dad had committed adultery with my mother. We never discovered the identity of the letter writer.

* * *

I broached the subject of the move to Devon during my next visit to New Malden. I asked Mum if she felt she was coping on her own. She admitted to being anxious all the time, especially at night. I'd tried to encourage her to occupy her days more constructively, but Mum didn't appear to be able to concentrate on anything. We'd walked together to the library to borrow a few books, but she couldn't read them. The television was constantly on, but was just a means of breaking the silence. She was unable to sit through a programme, always restless, continuously on the move as she trailed, without purpose, from room to room.

Mum had always claimed to be deeply in love with my father, but didn't display grief in the accepted sense. I know we all deal with the death of a loved one in different ways, but Mum didn't appear to mourn her loss, or even talk about Dad. She was emotionally shrivelled, except for anger, agitation and an inability to engage with life.

The other aspect that concerned me was my mother's weight loss. She prepared meals when I stayed with her, but I doubted whether she bothered to cook for herself when alone, although she declared that she did. My mother had certainly developed a sweet tooth, especially for a certain butterscotch sweet wrapped in gold paper. These wrappers would be located in the oddest places, folded into neat strips, but never thrown away. She now only had the use of three digits on the left hand. Her little finger and ring finger were always bent over into her palm because, underneath those fingers, she stashed more gold wrappers and would carry them around for hours.

***

Bob and I found a suitable bungalow in a cul-de-sac estate about two hundred yards from my home in Bideford, on the other side of a main road. It was tastefully decorated and compact, with a conservatory and a well laid out, easy-care garden, complete with fishpond. We brought Mum down to see it and to have a short holiday with Bob and his family. She didn't go into raptures over it exactly, but after a short period of deliberation, Mum informed us that she'd make the move. The implication was that this was for our benefit, which I guess, in many ways, it was.

I returned with my mother to New Malden, the offer having been made on the bungalow and accepted. As it was the school holidays, Jake and a friend of his came too. I thought we could combine sorting out some more of the never-ending rubbish and putting the house on the market with a bit of rest and relaxation, maybe a spot of sightseeing in London.

We took the slow train from Exeter to Waterloo. I've always thought of it as a more scenic route, and it provided a quaint trolley service that swayed its way through the carriages, offering drinks and snacks. It meant that nobody had to leave their seat, except for the toilet. Decidedly preferable to the scrum of the Penzance to Paddington train.

Mum seemed relaxed, acting the clown with the two boys. They were trying to teach her a card game. She made a big play of not being able to understand the rules, making obvious and hilarious mistakes which kept the boys amused for a good portion of the journey. I looked on and wondered. Was this a genuine comedy routine or an elaborate cover-up because, in reality, she had no idea what the game was all about?

We caught the main line train from Waterloo to Motspur Park, the same journey I'd covered so many times during the last few months. Mum lived fifteen minutes walk from the station and normally I would have walked it, but because of the amount of luggage we had between us, I decided to get a taxi. I left my little posse in the car park of the Earl Beatty pub, while I crossed the road to the phone box. It took five minutes at the most and I was within sight and shouting distance.

Whether it was because I hadn't prepared her beforehand about getting a taxi, or because she'd momentarily been left on her own with two eleven-year-old boys, I don't know. In those five minutes, she'd revved herself up into a state of hysteria, bordering on a major tantrum. We had to wait ten minutes, it felt more like an hour, with Mum getting more agitated by the second.

'We could have walked it by now,' she said.

'All the taxis will be busy, it's rush hour.'

'Why did you have to get a taxi? I'm quite capable of walking.'

The taxi pulled up in the road, alongside the car park. I directed the boys to pick up their bags and turned my attention to gathering the remaining luggage and my mother. But my mother was already trotting towards the taxi, oblivious to the bags scattered around us and the two-foot high wall between her and the car. She fell over the wall, smack flat onto the concrete.

The taxi driver leapt into action, as did the boys and passers-by, to retrieve this elderly lady from the ground.

In that moment, I was consumed with every emotion except the one I should have felt. Compassion. What I did feel, in those few seconds when chaos reigned and I stood looking on, was anger at her apparent stupidity, embarrassment that she should be the cause of this fiasco and fear she'd done some serious damage that would necessitate more time and care from her overstressed only daughter. The moment passed, and I resumed the role of concerned parent and entered into the fray.

Remarkably, she was unhurt except for minor grazes and dented pride, and we managed the remainder of the journey without further trauma.

The visit was an unexpected success assisted by a spell of good weather. I cleared out the shed and dumped most of the contents, except for a few obscure bits that I couldn't identify, which I transferred to the garage. My brother had expressed the desire to clear the garage himself as there were items, such as ladders and tools, which he felt were worth keeping.

The house was valued, put on the market and we had the first viewing, all within that week. That viewing led to an offer well below the asking price, but was accepted after procrastination, debate, false hope of a better offer and fear that we might lose the buyer we had. I even managed to take the boys to the South Kensington Natural History and Science Museums. A very productive week.

***

Bob had a very close relationship with his father. I think it had developed over the years since I'd moved away and after Bob and Marie had produced two children.

Dad was very fond of his granddaughters. In his latter years he'd mellowed and was the ideal granddad. The two girls still argue now, twenty years after his death, over who was Granddad's favourite but I genuinely believe he loved them both equally and without reservation.

That's why I was surprised at his decision not to move to Devon when Bob transferred his family there in 1983. Charlotte was only five years old and Carly, eighteen months younger, when the family relocated. I thought at the time that Dad was too set in his ways to contemplate the upheaval and I still think that was partly the reason. But did the early onset of dementia in my mother's life deter Dad from making the move away from all that was familiar to her?

***

About eighteen months after Bob's move to Devon, our parents financed a holiday at Butlin's in Minehead. Bob and Marie were running a busy pub in partnership with another couple and were unable to take the week off, so it was going to be the grandparents, Jake, Carly, Charlotte and me. I had a vague, unsubstantiated sense of foreboding but suppressed it. After all, Mum had always been a capable and inventive carer of young children.

Bob took the children and me to meet the parents at Minehead and left us to it. It soon became obvious that it was five children and me. I was decision maker, lawgiver and law enforcer. Not a position I was comfortable with.

Bob had always accused me of being too strong on the discipline front. The fact that Jake would sit at the dining table in the company of adults without having to be shouted at, nagged, bribed or embarrassing his parents, Bob saw as proof that I was too controlling. My argument was that good training meant I didn't embarrass us both in a public situation because Jake knew my expectations and was eager to rise to the occasion. That was until he was in the company of his loud, extrovert, mutinous older cousins and grandparents who refused to condemn outrageous behaviour. A nightmare.

I was exasperated with my mother who appeared unable to play any constructive role in this holiday. I'd already anticipated my father's "laissez faire" attitude. Dad, post retirement, was not high-functioning outside his comfort zone, but he certainly flourished at Butlin's fairground.

I've never been able to endure roundabout type rides without throwing up and most of Butlin's rides were of that persuasion. It was up to Granddad, or the kids were in danger of starting a full scale, three-pronged strop.

It was the waltzer ride that was his eventual undoing. Dad had taken Charlotte, aged six and by far the most daring of the three, onto the waltzer. He visibly turned green after the first two circuits. As he passed us for the fifth time, his face had become set in a taut grimace, which might have been construed, by the casual onlooker, as a smile denoting exhilaration. I knew differently. This was a man about to lose the entire contents of his stomach, and the only thing preventing this ignominious act were his false teeth, clenched together to form a dam. Charlotte bounced off the waltzer with her usual effervescence. Dad staggered off in the direction of our chalet, his complexion by then corpse grey.

Charlotte was high on life. It was impossible to dilute, even when I almost drowned her on the enclosed water flume. To be more accurate, I landed on top of her as we hurtled at a heart stopping rate out of the flume into the pool. We both went under the water. I couldn't get my footing. In a state of panic I failed to release my grip on Charlotte, thus holding her under. The pool's lifeguard waded in and hauled us out, Charlotte still laughing. I was mortified by the public exhibition and my near-death experience.

From my point of view, the holiday was a disaster from start to finish, not aided by the weather. It was the last week in May, wet and freezing. I think the children probably enjoyed it. Jake totally succumbed to peer pressure, and all three ignored any attempts at child control. I gave up, except where actual life and limb were at risk. Needless to say, Bob was told that there wouldn't be a repeat performance. I wasn't designed for overseeing a family of five children. My maternal instincts couldn't stretch that far.

***

By 1989, Dad's sister, also called Joan, was exhibiting symptoms of Alzheimer's disease. I recall going to visit her at Dad's request to see how, or if, she was managing on her own. While he kept his sister busy going through paperwork and bills, I did a quick reconnoitre of the bathroom and kitchen. Both showed signs of neglect, but more telling was the emptiness of the kitchen. Except for the usual appliances, there was nothing on the work surfaces, not even a stray crumb, and the cupboards, fridge and freezer were sparsely stocked. It was obvious that if she was eating properly, it wasn't at home.

Under subtle interrogation, it transpired that Joan was living on a diet of cheese, nuts and apples. Nothing cooked, but did that matter? Not ideal, but it was a trade off allowing her to continue living in her own home with the support of family and friends.

Dad managed to keep her afloat until his death. Without the anchor and support that he'd given his sister, she soon became too much of a liability left on her own and was moved to Yorkshire to live with her daughter, Pam, who would prove to be one of my main sources of support in the years to come.

***

These were the early signs of Joan's descent into Alzheimer's during the ten years leading up to my father's death. She changed from an outgoing, capable mother and wife, to someone regressing into uncharacteristic childishness, construed by me as attention-seeking behaviour. She appeared to lose interest in the day to day activities of her family and became increasingly neurotic and self-obsessed. Her ability to perform tasks that had been second nature to her, decreased and her physical clumsiness increased. It led to the deterioration in my own relationship with my mother, yet the changes had developed so slowly and with such subtlety that I didn't recognise the implications. However, I was convinced that without her husband, Joan would have difficulty living on her own.

PART 2

Chapter Four

Two days before the move to Bideford, Bob and I arrived at New Malden to pack up the contents of the house ready for the removal company. Mum was going to stay with Bob and Marie for a week to give us a chance to get her new home up and running. It would have been preferable to have moved her first, but she had other ideas. Mum wanted to supervise the clearance of the house she'd shared with Dad for the last forty-five years or more. I hadn't anticipated how much time it would take to wade through the collected dross, with my mother as self-appointed overseer of operations.

There wasn't much furniture to move and it was mostly chipboard and fitted, or fit for the dump. Mum insisted that the dining-room suite and sideboard must go with her, even though she'd professed to hate them because they were relics of Dad's first marriage. It was the books, records, tapes, old toys, Christmas decorations and tins of photographs that threatened to consume time we didn't possess, all of which she felt compelled to root through piece by piece.

The removal company arrived from Devon a day early, which threw me into a state of flux. They'd completed a move nearby and it wasn't worth their going all the way back to Bideford. Having recovered from the shock I was so delighted, I could have kissed them. Bob and the three musketeers took over downstairs and methodically packed the lot. Meanwhile I kept my mother busy upstairs, distracting her every time she voiced the desire to go and check that the workers were earning their wages, which was every ten minutes.

Marie, who'd been staying with her sister nearby, transported Mum from the area she was unlikely to see again, to Bideford. I'd anticipated a tearful departure, but it was notable that she displayed no emotion whatsoever. On the journey home, Marie took a wrong route and had to make a lengthy detour to get back on track. Mum's response to this was that her daughter-in-law wasn't to expect petrol money for the extra mileage she'd clocked up. Not that anyone had ever mentioned charging her for the journey.

With Mum safely ensconced at Bob's, the move into the bungalow in Bideford went smoothly. It was a small, secure estate populated by the elderly, with no children rampaging in the street causing unnecessary stress and anxiety to the residents. Her neighbours were friendly, especially considering that their son and daughter-in-law had wanted to buy the bungalow, but were unable to meet the purchase price.

***

Life dropped into a routine. I was still working part-time in a nearby nursing home and popped in to see my mother every day. From the start it was obvious that certain skills were beyond her, but tasks that she'd always performed, cooking, housework, shopping, were still within her range of ability. She was physically fit for a seventy-three-year-old and was still able to walk the best part of two miles into the town and back again. Mum wouldn't use the bus and driving the car was, by now, not an option. Gardening and decorating had been my father's domain and she was unable to learn new skills, however basic. I picked up the shortfall.

Mum agreed to keep the car, but relinquish her licence. It proved invaluable. I only had a motor scooter and was denied use of my husband's car for anything other than the weekly shopping. This new freedom meant I could take her on short trips and supermarket shopping once a week. We even managed a five day holiday together during her first year in Bideford, in the summer of 1995. We went to Harrogate, care of a coach company. It wasn't an overwhelming success. I hadn't realised how people with the onset of dementia cling to the familiar and can function reasonably well in the early stages, provided routine and well-constructed patterns remain in their lives. Remove all that and chaos ensues.

***

Mum became anxious from the start of the journey and clung to me like sticky weed. She was incapable of making any decisions for herself, even about what to eat. Every mealtime she selected the same item from the menu that I'd chosen for myself. This may have been because she could no longer read with comprehension, although Mum could still recognise words. I tried reading the menu to her, but she was unable to retain the information.

'I'll have the same as you,' she said.

My mother couldn't find her way around the hotel, so I had to escort her everywhere. If I left her on her own in the bedroom we shared, she would become panic stricken. The nights were an interesting glimpse into the future. I'd given Mum the bed next to the en suite bathroom, the door to the outside corridor was on the opposite wall with my bed between her and freedom. Every night I was woken up by my disoriented mother going to the bathroom. The problem was, Mum would make for the outside door instead of the bathroom door, by the most direct route, scrambling over my bed and me.

We did have some pleasant outings, though when your parent has become a child, it certainly brings its own unique problems. Crossing roads was treacherous in an alien environment. All road sense had disappeared. My suggestion that she take my arm was met with a belligerent outburst.

'I'm not a child!'

I walked on ahead of her, embarrassed by her top volume protest in the middle of York. The sudden shout and the crashing of metal on tarmac spun me round. An irate cyclist was lifting her bike from the road while berating

Mum for walking out in front of her. No people were injured in this episode.

Dad's sister lived not far from Harrogate with her daughter, Pam. One of the reasons that I'd chosen this part of Britain for a holiday was the opportunity to meet up with them. I arranged a rendezvous in the lounge of our hotel. It was a convivial evening. My aunt had progressed further than my mother down the Alzheimer's route, which had become an obvious issue some six years earlier. I was interested to note any signs for future reference, especially as this holiday had shown me that the problems with Mum were definitely not going away. The two Joans were snuggled together on the settee, chatting and laughing, oblivious to their surroundings. It was lovely to watch, but heart-wrenching too. These two women, both struggling to keep a hold on reality, immersed in the familiar past. I wanted to cry. Pam knew how I felt, we'd been in touch frequently during the previous eighteen months, comparing notes and advice. When they left I felt a sense of abandonment.

As soon as we returned home, I made an appointment with Mum's GP. I went without her because I needed to talk about my fears for my mother. The doctor was a bear of a man in his early thirties, with an easy manner and gentleness that I found comforting. I'd warmed to him when we'd been introduced on the day I'd taken her to register at the health centre, so it was an easy transfer to make when my own doctor left with ill health and I had to choose an alternative GP. More importantly, Mum liked him and as she was beginning to display wariness of men or, in the case of my husband, vicious hatred, her trust in the doctor was a bonus.

He listened, while I attempted to explain about my mother's inability to learn new skills or to hold onto the skills she once had and my concern about her increased memory loss, anxiety and childlike behaviour. He nodded slowly in acknowledgement of a problem revealed, but explained that it would be difficult, at this stage, to be certain of the cause.

'Alzheimer's is the major cause of dementia, but by no means the only one. Joan has a history of high blood pressure so she could be experiencing Transient Ischemic Attacks, small blood clots in the brain, which come and go. The symptoms can include confusion and memory loss along with temporary weakness of the limbs, slurred speech, sleepiness and non-response to external stimuli. The list goes on.'

I watched as he drew me a graph.

'Joan will experience a dip in her well-being when she has a TIA, but the symptoms will usually plateau or even disappear to some degree, if not completely.'

He drew a long horizontal line, turned the line downwards and then into an upward curve.

'However, if it's Alzheimer's disease, the line will continue to go down, the symptoms will get progressively worse and her ability, across the board, will become impoverished as more and more of the brain is destroyed.'

I already knew the end result. I'd worked in that field of care for too long not to know.

'How long?' I asked, in a tone that conveyed the bleakness I felt.

'I wish I had a crystal ball, but it depends on age, when it started and what the cause is. If it's TIAs, with the right medication Joan could go on for years at this level, with dips every now and then and a very slow overall deterioration in her condition.'

He keyed relevant details onto his computer.

'I'm making another appointment for Joan, to take some blood tests, check her blood pressure and we'll need a urine sample, just to rule out any other possible causes.'

I nodded in silent assent and we both stood, to signal my departure. He grasped my hand in a dry handshake.

'Try not to worry, this may not get any worse for a long time.'

I left, hoping for the best, but fearing the worst. I'd seen no other symptoms to explain a TIA except the memory loss and confusion, which were on a downward line on the graph with no upturns.

**

I was toying with the idea of changing my job. Being with Mum for extended periods, then working with the elderly, was too much exposure to the end of life processes. An incident at work made my decision for me. At a staff meeting, a member of staff was shouted at by the boss and owner of the home. It was likely that she was deserving of the dressing-down he gave her, but not the public bully-boy tactics he employed. I walked out of the meeting, upset by his outburst.

Events spiralled out of control after my exit and led to the girl handing in her notice. She subsequently went before an industrial tribunal, claiming constructive dismissal and I was subpoenaed as a witness to my boss's behaviour at the staff meeting. She lost her case. I was left feeling uncomfortable every time I came face to face with my employer who, in fairness to him, had never raised his voice or been anything but pleasant to me before this event, or after it. But it was the push I needed.

My mother's blood and urine tests had all come back clear and after another visit to the GP she'd been prescribed medication to reduce her anxiety levels. Mum seemed to be enjoying the summer months and appeared less agitated, so I decided to apply for a factory job, cleaning and packing cosmetic pencils. I thought we might both be able to cope.

I know many people decry factory work as mindless and boring but I enjoyed it. After a few weeks I was "promoted" to machine operator on a thumping, clanking monster that stamped the pencils with the logo of whichever company they were destined for. Take your eyes off that beast for a second and it would run out of foil or perform some other spiteful act and hundreds of pencils would be mutilated beyond salvaging. Boring it wasn't.

But Mum's condition continued to deteriorate. Her lack of intelligible speech was proving to be a major problem, coupled with her declining memory. Two events led to the reassessment of my wisdom in taking on a full-time job.

I always went to see my mother after I'd fed my family. This particular evening, she was subdued and winced when getting out of her chair. It transpired that she'd walked into town that day and had fallen outside Boots, the high street chemist. Several people came to her aid and sat her down in the chemist while the pharmacist dressed her cut and grazed knees. The accident wasn't serious, just one of the numerous falls she was prone to. More worrying was that well-meaning people offered to drive her home, but she was unable to tell them where she lived. My mother had forgotten her address.

She could be plausible, smile on cue and articulate set phrases in the appropriate places, which meant the average person would have no idea that Mum had a problem. But what was going to happen if she took a wrong turning into a street she didn't know? How would my mother ask for directions? Worse still, what if she forgot the way home altogether? I thought of different ways around the problem. An SOS necklace with all her details enclosed within the medallion. A card with her address and my contact details, kept inside her purse. Mum refused to wear the necklace and protested at the card idea, so I doubted if it would remain in her bag for long.

A few days later, on a Saturday afternoon, I answered the insistent ringing of the doorbell to find my next-door neighbour standing before me on the step with my mother beside her. Mum had been wandering up and down the road looking for my house. She was in a distressed state and couldn't remember exactly which house I lived in. It has to be said that she didn't visit often because she heartily disliked my husband and had announced, within his hearing, that she'd like to stick a knife in his back. Under the circumstances, I had to presume that this was a mission of importance.

It transpired that Mum couldn't open her front door.

'The thing won't do the door!' she shrieked.

My mother was frustrated and angry with herself and me. I feared that she'd forgotten how to unlock the front door. With a heavy heart, I escorted her back to the bungalow and was almost relieved to find that the Yale lock had developed a fault and indeed the key wouldn't open the door.

She felt vindicated and was suddenly quite chirpy as we returned to my house to phone the locksmith. He arrived three hours later, having spent most of his day at a nearby notorious housing estate, fixing the locks and doors damaged by the Friday night drunken domestic disputes. He shot off the old lock and fitted a new Yale lock and charged me forty pounds. Job done, or so I thought. I gave it no further consideration until one night, some days later.

On my habitual evening visits during the following week, each time I put the key in the lock to open the door, it would just push open without turning the key. Mum was usually fastidious about locking herself indoors. I didn't make too much of it, after all it was summer and the evenings were still warm and doused with late sunlight when I went over to the bungalow.

She would come to the door to say goodbye when I left, and I'd remind her to lock it, as I escaped down the garden path. As the week progressed, Mum became jittery with anxiety. I couldn't understand what was wrong. She was trying to tell me, but no longer had the vocabulary to convey the problem, and I was too busy berating her for the folly of leaving her door unlocked.

Finally the penny dropped. My mother had forgotten how to use the button on the lock to release or hold back the catch. The lock itself was identical to the old one, except for the colour. Five days earlier Mum had experienced no problems using the lock. It seemed that the difference in colour rendered it as something alien in her mind and therefore wiped the instruction on how to work a Yale lock from her brain.

Time to call in little brother. We discussed the options and decided that it would be best to remove the Yale and replace it with a simple lock and key. It would be a safer option. She was already using this type of lock on her back door, so we hoped she would be able to operate this one, plus it would negate the likelihood of accidentally locking herself out.

From that point on, Joan's life started to unravel at a frightening pace. Every day would throw up new problems to be thought through and overcome. It was obvious that her level of care would have to increase. I handed my notice in at the factory. I'd been there for three months.

***

I have to pay homage to Mum's sister, Olive, and her husband, Dennis. Since my father's death they'd been very supportive. They took her to stay with them in Birmingham for a couple of weeks that first Easter and for the first two Christmases. This was a gratefully received gift to me and to her sister, at the start.

Those periods of time when Mum was with Olive were respite for me, a time to re-energise. Therefore I was delighted when Olive said that she and Dennis would like to come to Bideford to stay for a week during the summer. Olive was a "doer". She didn't stand on the perimeter thinking, *should I or not? Will I upset anyone if I do?* She got stuck in, gathered up the reins and took over. Just what I needed. I had the week off, Mum was taken out and about, and Olive and Dennis had a short holiday, with free accommodation, in glorious Devon. Result. Though I wouldn't have described living with my mother for a week as a holiday, I was grateful.

***

Coming up to her second Christmas as a widow, my mother was grumbling about what presents to get for Bob, his family and Ray and Jake. As I don't celebrate Christmas, I was being less than helpful. My suggestion was money, and then they could all get what they wanted. Anyway I hadn't got a clue what was high on the wish list for teenage girls and a silent husband.

She begrudgingly conceded that this was probably the best idea and rooted in her purse for some five pound notes, in order to distribute one for each person. I protested that she could afford to be a little more generous, especially as she never gave them anything on any other occasion, apart from birthdays. This had little to do with dementia. My parents had always lacked spontaneity in the giving department. An argument ensued and I stomped off.

I told myself that, as far as I was concerned, she could do what she liked, I'd given her my opinion. If she chose to ignore it, so be it.

A couple of weeks later Mum broached the subject again, as if the previous conversation had never taken place. She'd decided to give everyone ten pounds each. She managed to write "love Nan", "love Mum" and "Joan" in the relevant cards and asked me to write names on the envelopes, which I did. She then proceeded to dole out the cash for each one. Mum handed me the money for the first recipient. *Ten* ten pound notes. This uncharacteristic spurt of generosity prompted a few questions from me. It transpired that she now thought a ten pound note was worth one pound.

A look in her handbag confirmed my suspicions. My mother had walked into Bideford and withdrawn five hundred pounds from the bank. She'd then walked around Bideford with the handbag, which was always going missing, just before Christmas, when opportunist thieves were on the lookout for demented little old ladies. I was just grateful that she'd no idea how to use a cash machine.

I was mid-diatribe, trying to explain to her the error of her ways, when the doorbell rang. It was my brother. I said nothing about the money, but Mum was visibly agitated and upset, so the story came out over a cup of tea, which resulted in another lecture from Bob.

'I think you'd better put the money in the bureau, apart from what you need now,' Bob advised.

But the five hundred pounds had disappeared. It wasn't in her bag, down the side of the settee she was sitting on, or under it.

'Where have you put it, Mum?' I asked.

Tears and denial were the only response. We turned the lounge upside down with no result. Bob left and I could tell by the set of his jaw that he wasn't a happy bunny. To keep having confirmation that your mother is losing her marbles is like surgical spirit in a raw wound and an unwelcome reminder that we shared some of her genes.

I continued the search, spreading the net, as you do, to the most unlikely places. My mother was wandering from room to room wringing her hands. The problem wasn't so much the mislaid money, it was here somewhere and would undoubtedly turn up sooner or later. But now she knew it was five hundred and not fifty pounds, she was distraught at its loss. I knew she wouldn't settle until it was found. The stash was eventually discovered under the mattress in her bedroom. I could only think that when Bob rang the doorbell and I went to open the door, she'd been stricken with panic and hurriedly squirrelled the money away in the traditional safe place.

That second Christmas in 1995 was the last one spent with Olive. By the third Christmas, Joan's deterioration was such that she was no longer able to cope with breaks in routine and unfamiliar situations increased her anxiety and disorientation. Her world was closing in.

Chapter Five

I decided to join a carer's group run by the Alzheimer's Society. We met on the last Monday evening in the month to listen to advice and insight imparted to us from guest speakers. Afterwards, we swapped useful tips and experiences over a cup of tea.

Through the group, two important factors came to light that hitherto nobody had mentioned. Mum was eligible for Attendance Allowance, which would help me financially, having given up work in order to provide her with the care she needed.

The other issue we were advised to think about, was the future. Bob and I needed to get Power of Attorney for when it all inevitably fell apart. The problem was that Joan had to appear, to the solicitor, as being of sound mind and that wouldn't bear close scrutiny. She also needed to be able to sign her own name, and her ability to do that was teetering on the point of oblivion.

We visited the solicitor without Mum as there was no point in raising his suspicions too far in advance. He advised us to apply for Joint Enduring Power of Attorney, which we initially agreed to, but then I read an article in the Alzheimer's Society's monthly news sheet. We should have been applying for Enduring Power of Attorney, jointly and severally, which meant that if either one of us became unable to fulfil our commitment as an attorney, the other one would automatically take over. Under the solicitor's guidance, if one of us could no longer act as an attorney, the Power of Attorney would become null and void. Joan's affairs would then have to be dealt with by the Court of Protection, an expensive and impractical alternative.

We informed the solicitor of the action he should have recommended. His failure to advise us correctly may have gone some way to his overlooking the fact that Mum was far from with it when she presented herself at his office. Anxiety had robbed her of speech, but she managed a whispered assent when asked if she understood what was taking place and if she was in agreement with it. Mum applied a shaky signature on the dotted line and that was that. It was another eighteen months before we needed to activate it.

These days Enduring Power of Attorney is called a Lasting Power of Attorney and all the forms can be downloaded from the Office of the Public Guardian web site, cutting out the cost of a solicitor. Not to be undertaken by the faint-hearted, but then what official form is?

***

I investigated the possibility of applying for Carer's Allowance, but it was only awarded if you were devoting thirty-five hours, or more, a week to caring for someone. That wasn't the case, at that time, so I couldn't submit a claim, even though the fragmented nature of the care I provided meant it was difficult to fit other employment into the time frame.

The forms to complete for Attendance Allowance were something else. I'd advise anyone, undergoing a similar procedure, to get help, one brain isn't sufficient. It's difficult enough to fill out a claim for yourself, but to answer the questions on behalf of someone who can no longer communicate their needs, while trying to anticipate the deterioration the next week will bring, was almost impossible. I completed the questions to the best of my ability, in the present rather than the unknown but predictable future. Joan was awarded Attendance Allowance at the lower rate, which meant that, technically, she was only in need of care during the daytime, not at night.

The forms needed to go to her GP for his ratification. I thought I'd take them in personally as he hadn't seen Mum for a few months and the details I was asking him to endorse, described a different lady to the one he thought he knew. The doctor listened sympathetically, as I updated him on my mother's decline.

'What I'd like to do,' he said, 'is to ask the consultant geriatrician to visit Joan at home to do an assessment. It will be more accurate done in a familiar environment.' He concentrated his gaze at his computer screen. 'Tell Joan its part of an MOT we give patients over a certain age.'

The consultant geriatrician arrived some two weeks later. I'd tried to play it down when broaching the subject of the visit with Mum but her anxiety levels were very acute. A man, especially a medical consultant, making a home visit was enough to put her into a complete tizzy.

My mother had, in the last decade, become something of a hypochondriac, seeking medical attention for one imagined illness after another. A personal visit from a consultant geriatrician was something to cherish rather than fear and certainly an occasion to dress up for.

When he arrived, it was enough to put me into tizzy mode and made me wish I'd made an effort to change out of my jogging bottoms and T-shirt. Talk about a Greek god. He filled the doorway with blond virility.

I left them to it. About an hour later he came into the kitchen to talk to me. Yes, there was a problem. No, he couldn't tell me the cause. It wasn't really relevant, the effects would be the same and her ability to function impaired on all levels. He'd like Joan to attend the Abbotsvale Centre, for one day a week. Abbotsvale was a specialist unit that dealt with dementia and cognitive impairment. The staff there would help to stimulate Joan's remaining memory, teach her some techniques to help her cope independently for longer, and monitor her progress or regression.

I remained with Mum after the Greek god had departed and talked her through what had just taken place and what would happen, as a result. I played down the cause of her memory loss, attributing her decline to all the changes that had taken place in her life recently. I was talking rubbish, but Mum's standard response was going to be to refuse to entertain the idea of going to Abbotsvale. I was going to have to sell this idea to her with diplomacy and determination.

The letter of confirmation came through some days later.

Well, I thought, *at least it's an outing that doesn't involve me, except as duty driver. It will give her something to talk to me about, and maybe she'll make a friend, who knows?*

Mum agreed to go with all the resistant attitude that I'd expected. By now the drugs she was taking for anxiety were doing their job, so it was more belligerence than fear, which I could deal with. Her stubbornness didn't tempt me to feel sorry for her and capitulate. I was determined that she was going to go, promising that if she hated it after a month she wouldn't have to go anymore. Mum needed to make a life for herself in Bideford and this could be a start. She agreed, not exactly with a good grace or willingness, but she went.

***

We got into the routine of the once a week trip to Abbotsvale. The staff were pleasant and Trish, her key worker, was a joy. I can't say that it improved my mother's cognitive function one iota, but it was a few hours that I could spend cleaning her bungalow, which by now was showing signs of her inability to perform even basic tasks.

Mum adamantly declared that she was quite capable of doing her own housework, and that she dusted every day, which she undoubtedly did. The problem was, she dusted the same bit, which never extended beyond the lounge. The kitchen was becoming a health hazard with accumulated dirt and out of date food. In the bathroom, the shower unit had developed it own eco system, living within a quagmire of soapy sludge. If my mother noticed that her home was being cleaned for her, she never let on, and I didn't mention it.

Her time at Abbotsvale was beneficial in other ways. My mother had, by nature, been a gregarious woman, a performer. Being with people lifted her spirits. She ate well when she returned home and was more animated and talkative. So, I reasoned, how could I extend the experience to broaden out her life a little more?

Trish said that Mum would be a good candidate for the local day centre. She suggested that I contact Social Services. The result was that Mum was offered one day a week. She would be picked up and returned home by their transport. That one day could be extended to two, if I could bring Joan to the day centre on the additional day. A small price to pay for the quality of life it would give to her and the extra freedom afforded to me. Again, I had the initial reluctance to overcome, but I stood firm, feeling like the parent sending her offspring to school for the first time.

She loved it. The centre overlooked Victoria Park, and had its own landscaped garden to sit in, when weather permitted. Mum even made a friend there, whose name I've long since forgotten, but I do remember that she was invited round to her new friend's flat for tea. This was a step too far. Joan wasn't, by then, able to sustain a one to one relationship without support. Still, it was giving her a life beyond her own four walls.

* * *

One of the reasons that Joan now found relationships difficult was the increased language problem. Words were disappearing from her vocabulary at an alarming rate. Sometimes the elusive word would be replaced with "the thing", "the whatsit" or "you know", which I invariably didn't. Increasingly, a completely inappropriate word would be substituted. These were starting to outnumber the meaningful ones, which resulted in speech that had the intonation of a normal conversation, but made no sense at all. Joan knew, in her head, what she wanted to say, it just wasn't coming out of her mouth. Somewhere between brain and lips the words were sabotaged. Understandably, her sense of frustration at herself and her bemused audience was often ill disguised.

Trish confirmed that my mother's communication skills were diminishing. She'd run some tests just to see how much meaningful vocabulary Mum had left. She was unable to remember the names for the majority of everyday objects shown to her in picture format. Sometimes, she would find an alternative, if inappropriate word, but many times nothing was forthcoming.

An interesting side issue emerged from this one to one session with Trish. My mother voiced her regret that she'd been unable to protect me against my father's temper. How she conveyed this information to Trish, I never thought to ask. Perhaps because I was so taken aback that it had troubled her for all these years. It was a subject that I don't recall ever discussing with Mum and certainly had never mentioned to Trish.

* * *

Before my mother moved to Bideford, she was still driving to her hairdresser once a week. How she accomplished this without killing herself or somebody else, I'll never know. I felt that it was important for her to continue her weekly visits to a salon, but on foot. There was a small hairdresser's salon about three hundred yards away from her bungalow. There was one snag, it was on the other side of the main road, but at the time I viewed this as an acceptable risk. After all, Mum had to cross the same road when she walked into town, and so far she'd survived unscathed.

The two hairdressers that worked in the salon very soon sussed out that there was a problem, and proved to be caring, beyond the call of duty. For the first year, my mother continued to be independent in this weekly ritual. On the rare occasion that she failed to turn up for her appointment, they would ring me. Usually it meant Mum was having a bad morning where she couldn't find anything, was unable to get herself dressed and just generally couldn't get it together. The mornings were her worst time, increasingly so as the dementia continued to strip Joan's brain of her ability to function.

The missed appointments and telephone calls from the salon gradually increased and were becoming the norm rather than the exception. It obviously couldn't continue so I changed her appointments to the afternoon, when Mum was usually more with it. If she was having a crazy day, I had all morning to get her ready. Then, the main road began to be problematic. I'd noticed that Mum would start the process of crossing a road but rarely reach the opposite footpath. Her trajectory would take her close to the kerb, but she would continue in her chosen direction in the gutter. Not a healthy pursuit. I made the decision to escort her to the hairdressers and pick her up an hour later. This extended the weekly appointment for a while longer, until two separate incidents occurred that marked the beginning of the end of this chapter of Joan's life.

One afternoon, the hairdresser rang to say that they were worried, because my mother had refused to wait for me to collect her and had stomped out of the shop in an agitated state. I hoped her unescorted departure from the salon was a one-off, knowing, of course, that it wouldn't be. Joan's anxiety and agitation levels were increasing generally, as her memory and her ability to make sense of her world were decreasing. She could no longer converse with people or relate to them as an adult. Joan was becoming more childlike, with a level of reasoning to match. She constructed her own version of events to fill in the gaps she didn't understand, or had forgotten. Even this inevitable work of faction couldn't be conveyed with any clarity.

'Confabulation,' the doctor explained during one of my visits to update repeat prescriptions for Mum.

He smiled mischievously, leaning back in his chair, legs outstretched and crossed at the ankles.

'I recall visiting a lovely old gentleman in hospital, who had dementia,' he said. 'He had a bed by the window with a view over the city, but was convinced he was on a cruise ship. He could even describe the views from his window as a port he knew well. You see, he couldn't make sense of where he was, but he needed to, so his brain constructed a reassuring scene to fit around the tiny bits that seemed familiar to him. That's confabulation.'

I could understand the making up of events to fill in the gaps, but seeing a whole different physical scene, I couldn't really grasp that. I wasn't even sure if it was a real word or condition, or the doctor's fanciful sense of humour. Real word or not, I was going to get a practical demonstration of the condition in the very near future.

***

The television, kettle and cooker were now the only appliances that Mum could still work for herself. Washing machine, central heating, stereo, shower, lighting. All gone. Even the transistor radio was too complicated for her to master. I was constantly retuning it into a programme, because she'd had fiddled with the radio, tuning into dead air then abandoning it, thinking she'd switched the radio off.

Mum could still answer the phone, but was, by now, unable to make calls, even though she had a list of single digit speed dial numbers by the phone. The complicated physical and thought processes required which we take for granted, between reading a number and waiting while the connection

33

is made, were now impossible to perform. It was heartbreaking.

***

The pressure of running two homes was beginning to tell. I was also desperate for somebody to talk to. I needed to air my concerns about ways to overcome the numerous problems thrown up by the dementia that were demolishing every aspect of my mother's life, physically, emotionally and mentally. I was on a permanent guilt trip, because I knew I was coming up short on the emotional support front. I was also crushed by my marital breakdown. I tried hard to suppress the pain and despair of it all so that Jake's life didn't become any more traumatic than it already was.

I'd started to wedge a chair under the handle of my bedroom door at night. Not that Ray had ever been physically aggressive towards me, but I felt there had to be a meltdown point. His behaviour was so freezingly unnatural, with never a word, a smile or a touch directed my way. If I spoke to him, he wouldn't even look at me. It was as if I didn't exist, except as an irritant. Like a trapped bluebottle fly which eventually, if it persists in buzzing, will be swatted.

***

I was walking over to Mum's bungalow just after lunch one midweek afternoon. The intention was to vacuum and change the bed linen before she came back from the day centre. I halted mid-stride as I heard the gut wrenching sound of an accident and turned around to see a motorbike on the ground about a hundred yards away. I ran back. As I got closer I could see a female body lying at the side of the road. I passed a man, who'd just emerged from a doorway, alerted by the sound of the crash. As I ran past, I shouted to him to call an ambulance, my heart racing with the exertion of the hundred yard dash and rising panic at the scene that was evolving before me.

The elderly lady lying spread-eagled with her head resting against the kerb had sustained terrible injuries. Her left leg had been virtually sliced off at the groin. I had the fleeting vision of a cooked chicken, with its leg falling away from the body. There was blood coming from her ears, but virtually none from her leg and although her eyes weren't closed, she was seeing nothing. She was unconscious or worse.

As I knelt beside her, trying unsuccessfully to find a pulse, a car pulled up. A couple ran over with a blanket. The woman with the blanket attempted to find a spark of life, but couldn't. By now several people had gathered, wanting to help, but not knowing how. The man from the house informed us that the ambulance and police were on their way, but I think, collectively, we thought it was too late, though nobody dared to put words to that thought.

The motorcyclist, whose bike was still lying in the middle of the road, was crying and shaking uncontrollably. Some of the onlookers tried to comfort him, listening to his version of events with sympathy and much stroking of his back. He'd just returned from Bude, having been to a successful job interview.

'There was nothing I could do,' he wept, 'she walked right out in front of me.'

He kept repeating this sentence like a mantra, as if it was somehow going to undo the carnage.

It appeared that the woman, loaded with shopping, had got off the bus at the bus stop on the other side of the road from where her body lay and had simply stepped off the kerb and in front of the bike. How else could it have happened? It was a straight length of highway. The impact had been so violent that it had thrown her from one side of the main road to the gutter on the opposite side. Her shopping now lay strewn across the tarmac, though her handbag had been retrieved and placed beside her. I decided, rightly or wrongly, to look for some identification so at least we had a name to reassure her with. We all thought she was beyond hearing, but we felt the need to keep talking to her.

I found her bus pass, complete with her photograph. My shock was compounded by the realisation that I knew her. Elizabeth lived next door but one to me, my son and her grandson were mates. I just hadn't recognised this crumpled, mutilated person lying lifeless, unseeing eyes gazing towards the sky, as my sprightly, smartly dressed, neighbour.

We waited. It was all we could do.

The rapid response paramedic arrived first, followed swiftly by ambulance and police. By then, the band of onlookers had gathered up the motorbike and shopping from the road. The police weren't best pleased. They'd wanted everything left where it had landed.

The road was immediately closed to traffic. The motorcyclist was escorted to the police car. My neighbour was gently lifted from the road and put into the ambulance. Ominously, it was fifteen minutes or so before it moved off.

The police wanted everyone who hadn't actually witnessed the accident to disappear and were none too polite about it. We all wanted to stay, a core of post apocalyptic survivors, huddled together, trying to make sense of it all. I attempted to approach one of the police officers to tell him that I knew Elizabeth, and I knew her daughter and where she worked. He was having none of it.

'Did you see the accident?' he asked.

'No, but…'

'We only want to talk to people who saw what happened here. If you didn't, please move on, you're obstructing a police investigation.'

I started to walk away and then the red mist descended. He was going to have this information whether he wanted it or not. I turned, went back and told him just that. Ungraciously, he accepted what I had to say, then I fled the scene and returned home.

Once behind closed doors I wept with unrestrained grief. I wept for my neighbour and her daughter, who was going to have to cope with the aftermath of this horrendous event. I wept for Mum, who crossed that road regularly, and I cried for myself, because I'd stockpiled these tears for months. The dam had burst. I didn't know if I could stop it up again. Eventually, I regained control. My eyes were so puffy, I was seeing through slits, mucus leaked from my nose. I was weak with despair and exhaustion that emanated from my bone marrow.

That evening I visited her daughter at her mother's house. Elizabeth had died before she'd reached the hospital. I wasn't surprised. I didn't give her daughter any details, just told her that I thought Elizabeth had died instantly and that she certainly hadn't suffered. If I'd been her daughter, it would have comforted me to have known that. One thing was certain, I wasn't going to risk my mother coming back from the hairdresser alone and crossing that main road anymore.

Chapter Six

Enter Jeremy, a hairdresser and a friend, who had his own salon in nearby Northam, too far away from home for Mum to make her escape without me. At a push, I could deliver her to the salon, shop in the nearby supermarket and return within the hour. It was a feasible plan.

We experienced a few teething problems with the new arrangement. Jeremy's customer base was predominantly the over sixties, and my mother didn't see herself as part of this age group anymore. She still wanted her hair styled in soft curls rather than the "one style fits all" that Jeremy adhered to. I had to employ some subtle diplomacy to try to encourage him to produce a looser style for this particular customer. I was quite encouraged that my mother still had an opinion about her appearance, even if it threatened to cause a rift at the birth of this business arrangement. It took several visits before she warmed to Jeremy, and bless him, he did his best to get back into her good books, but her hair style never quite regained the girlish look she desired.

It was a workable solution to drop my mother at Jeremy's and then shop, while his version of a youthful style was being constructed. Mum and I had been doing the weekly shop together, but it'd become such a stressful event that I'd begun to dread it. Compiling the list and getting Mum ready were painfully time-consuming.

Keeping tabs on her in the supermarket was a challenge, she still had the speed of a whippet, but I had to ensure that we went through the checkout together because, by now, Mum had no idea about money and its worth and was unable to do anything constructive with a bank card.

Then there was the dreaded supermarket trolley. Having made it in one piece as far as the car park and transferred the shopping into the car, Joan would insist on returning the trolley to the designated area. If I refused to relinquish it, she would throw a tantrum at top volume, so I invariably caved in. The problem was that even if we were parked right next to the trolleys, Joan would return it and then take off in completely the opposite direction from the parked car. No amount of shouting, horn beeping, jumping up and down, and flailing my arms in the air like a demented marionette would divert her from her chosen route. Sometimes I'd just stand and watch her, wondering where this was all going to end and willing her to walk under the wheels of a bus. Then the guilt would kick in and I'd take retrieval action.

The cracks were beginning to show. I popped into the health centre for the regular blood pressure check required before renewing my prescription for hormone replacement therapy. The nurse asked me to return for another test the following day. The next day produced the same result. My blood pressure was unacceptably high which meant a visit to the doctor before there was any possibility of more HRT.

My doctor looked at me with an air of discernment, which convinced me that he suspected I was withholding vital information. In a sense that was true, but I never knew where to start, it was easier not to say anything. Once the floodgates were open, when and where would the outpouring stop? I knew I was a mess.

'I think you're depressed,' he said, composing his face to reflect sympathy. 'Do you ever have thoughts of harming yourself?'

I tried the flippant approach.

'I did have this fleeting thought on the A39. Mum was throwing one of her tantrums in the passenger seat. We were behind a tractor and trailer, and I did think that if I put my foot down on the accelerator and crashed into the back of the trailer, it would hopefully finish us both off, but I wouldn't really have done it.'

He nodded sagely, raised one eyebrow above the rim of his glasses and waited.

'I'm not suicidal,' I protested, 'but I'm always angry. Sometimes I have to abandon my trolley in the supermarket because I need to get out. I can't stand the noise and the people. I want to take a machine gun to everyone in there.'

There it was, out in the open, I wasn't coping anymore. The tears started, I was losing control and I hadn't got a tissue. The doctor handed me a box of tissues as he informed me that he was going to prescribe antidepressants.

'I think your raised blood pressure is due to stress, anxiety and depression,' he said. 'You've been carting round this wheelbarrow full of bricks for a long time now. Someone has chucked in one more than you can handle, and you're in danger of dropping the lot. Let's try this and I'll see you in four weeks.'

Armed with antidepressants and HRT tablets, I left.

The drug prescribed was Paroxetine. For me, it was a life saver, once I'd survived the first month. Three weeks after I started taking the antidepressants, I hit a brick wall. Twenty-four hours when I felt too exhausted to move my eyes, never mind the rest of me.

The overall effect of the drug was to bubble wrap me. I ceased to have any deep emotions about anything, good or bad. It robbed me of a large chunk of personality, but it wasn't a bad place to be when struggling with two major crises. A wrecked marriage and a demented mother. Plus all the problems that were cropping up daily as my mother's condition continued to decline.

***

My mother was still taking antidepressants, but continued to exhibit anxiety when life didn't adhere to a rigid routine. When she first came to live in Bideford, we would visit different places and still did, but the list was getting shorter.

When we went out, it had to be the same few destinations or her anxiety levels shot through the roof. It was obvious that she was out of her depth and eager to return home. If we went for a cup of coffee in town, it had to be the same café. If we fancied a Hockings ice cream we could only purchase cones from the van outside Victoria Park in Bideford, or next to the slipway at Westward Ho!

Hockings vans are dotted all over North Devon, such is the popularity of their clotted cream ice cream, but Mum would only devour a cornet bought from these two places. The upshot was that this limited list of familiar places had to be visited frequently or they became unfamiliar and had to be crossed off the list. The theatre had met with this fate.

During her first year in Devon, we went to the ballet at the Queen's Theatre in Barnstaple. It's a small theatre and it was ballet performed with recorded music. Personally, I found the sound of the dancers' shoes tap tapping across the stage an irritating distraction, but Mum loved it. She sat riveted to her seat, totally immersed in the performance.

I didn't have the opportunity to repeat the theatre experience until near the end of her second year in Bideford. By then, of course, it was on the list headed Unfamiliar Places to Avoid, only I hadn't worked all this out at that time.

We went to see the Glen Miller band, not *the* Glen Miller obviously, but an upmarket tribute band. I thought it would appeal to Mum, music from her era to excite familiar memories of a period in her life that hadn't yet totally disappeared into the mist of dementia. She remembered nothing of the first visit to the Queen's Theatre, and became agitated when confronted with the throng in the foyer. I thought she would calm down once seated, but she didn't.

It was an experience similar to sitting next to a bored, truculent toddler. All social graces expected of an adult had gone. Joan was constantly on the fidget, coat on, coat off, twisting round in the seat to inspect the people behind, turning out her handbag into her lap and onto the floor, looking for what? She'd no idea. Eventually, I snatched coat and bag from her and growled at her to sit still. Her response was exactly what you'd expect from a terrible two-year-old.

'I'm not a child!' she shrieked, above a somewhat lengthy drum solo.

I cringed, sank low in my seat and thrusted coat and bag back into her lap. She continued her antics throughout the entire performance, which seemed endless.

***

My mother's anxiety had recently spilled over into her home environment, which was disconcerting, because up to now she'd appeared quite settled in her bungalow. I let it pass for a few days, but her agitation levels remained high and she was quite distressed at times. I tried a bit of probing to find out if there was any solid foundation for her evident apprehension.

'There's a girl and she's got my clothes,' Mum stated.

This sentence came out as clear as a bell, as if it'd been rehearsed and stored, ready for the appropriate moment to tell me. I wasn't sure if she was being serious or trying to make a joke. She was serious.

Mum was convinced that there was a young girl, early teens perhaps, who was putting on her clothes, prancing around tauntingly in front of her, then running away. I sat with her trying to reason it through and although she agreed it couldn't be so and must all be in her imagination, I got the feeling that this was being said more to appease me than out of conviction on her part.

During the next few days there was evidence that Mum was avoiding the bedroom and sleeping on the settee. I took her into the bedroom. We sat on the edge of the bed together, as she tried to talk me through the experience of living with an adolescent thief.

The girl only appeared in the bedroom and apparently lived in the mirror fronted wardrobe. She flaunted herself in front of my mother, dressed in these stolen clothes, but when approached she would disappear into the wardrobe, only to reappear at another time. On one level, Mum knew that this was bizarre and unlikely, but how else could she explain the evidence of her own eyes? I promised her that I'd get it sorted. The only problem was — how? I went home, leaving Mum relieved that she'd handed the problem over to me.

During the evening I pondered this dilemma. What was going on? Obviously this wasn't a real girl, so what was happening? I spoke to Trish the next day, at Abbotsvale.

'Delusions,' she said. 'Joan is seeing something that doesn't exist. It's known that delusions can take many forms, but are common to people with dementia.'

I thought of my cousin, Pam. Her mother also had dementia and Pam and I were in frequent contact, bolstering each other up. Her mother was about five years ahead of mine down the dementia route. She would see children in her bedroom, not always welcome visitors, so she kept a supply of sweets in her room, to bribe them into leaving when asked to do so.

For Mum's sake this was a problem that had to have a solution. My mother was afraid to be in her own home and that wasn't an acceptable situation. I mulled over what the doctor had told me about confabulation versus Trish's delusion theory. I had a few theories of my own but I needed to run them by somebody else first before I acted on them. A conference with my brother was high on the agenda.

I had a gut feeling that this was confabulation at work. I felt that my mother was responding to her own reflection, but she was, for want of a more appropriate term, growing down. She saw herself in the mirror as a young girl. That tied in with her day to day behaviour which was becoming very childlike. Because her brain still acknowledged, on some level, that she was a seventy-something lady, she saw her own reflection as a stranger, someone who shouldn't be there. As Mum moved, in panic and anger, towards this reflection, to confront this brazen hussy, the girl disappeared. This, I reasoned, was either because the image, close up, became her own again or because Mum's attempt to chase the girl out of the bedroom meant that this spectre moved out of the reflective range and disappeared.

I sat on the edge of her bed, looking into the mirror. It was a feasible explanation. The mirror took up most of one wall because they were actually mirrored sliding doors to a built in wardrobe space. The only other feature on that wall was the door to the hallway. To me, it explained why Mum assumed that the girl was living in the wardrobe. If one of the mirrored doors was slightly open, at the bedroom door end, which it often was, the reflected area would cease there and the girl would seem to disappear into the wardrobe. It made perfect sense to me.

Bob looked at me incredulously as I explained my theory, but was at a loss to provide an alternative explanation. He immediately, as men do, looked for a solution. The obvious one was to remove the mirrors, but that wasn't going to be practical in terms of time, disposal and replacement. The other option was to cover the mirrors.

In true children of Blue Peter style, we decided that sticky backed plastic was a quick, cost effective and reversible solution. I purchased some rolls with a pretty pink pattern. Together we tackled the task while Mum was at the day centre. I have to say, it wasn't quite the easy option we'd envisaged. To cover that amount of glass, without huge bubbles appearing all over the place, was nigh on impossible, but we made a halfway decent stab at it. We left a small strip of mirror down the middle, which gave Mum a full length image of herself, but not the full width. If that proved to be a problem, we could cover that too.

It worked. I couldn't believe we'd found a remedy so easily. Joan accepted the cover-up and her restricted image didn't appear to pose a problem. If only all the difficulties waiting in the wings to bombard us were as easily resolved.

***

Christmas 1996 was the third Christmas since Dad's death, but the first that my mother was to spend in her bungalow at Bideford instead of with Olive and Dennis. Of course, the day centre and Abbotsvale were closed until after the New Year, although both places had their own version of a Christmas party. Whether or not she enjoyed the festivities, I'd no idea. By the time she returned home, it'd all been forgotten. I stayed with my mother on Christmas Day.

While Mum had been in Birmingham, I'd been using her home as my bolthole for the previous two Christmases. By now, her world had shrunk so much that it would have been too stressful for her to leave home for any length of time, and her increasing dislike of men had extended to Olive's husband as well as mine.

I'd been informed that after the Christmas break, Mum would be losing her Saturday slot at the day centre. The client base was changing from the elderly to clients with physical disabilities. Joan was beginning to find Saturdays difficult to cope with anyway. For some reason she was becoming distressed and reluctant to go there. They were a more able client group than the Monday crowd and I thought she may be out of her depth. Or perhaps she had taken a dislike to one of the staff or clients. Who knows? Extracting meaningful information was almost impossible now and conclusions were based on a high percentage of guesswork.

Mum wasn't at all upset at losing the Saturday, I was the one who found it difficult to accept. How long, I wondered, before the Monday session would prove too much for her, and then what?

***

There was no doubt that Joan was losing brain cells at an alarming rate. There were no longer easy solutions to the problems. I'd spent two days locating a smell that stank like faeces. I'd surreptitiously checked out her underwear, while supervising her shower, no problem there. I scoured the bungalow for suspicious stains and found nothing out of the ordinary, but the aroma lingered on.

On the third day of sniffing my way round her home like an obsessive bloodhound, I had occasion to open Mum's handbag to put money in her purse for the day centre. I was now in charge of finances since the Christmas five hundred pound debacle. There it was, in all its glory, a ball of human excrement, neatly wrapped in a tissue. My mother had obviously forgotten that she'd squirrelled this prize item away, and to be honest, I didn't see the point of broaching a subject that was past and obviously forgotten. It appeared that her olfactory senses were going the same way as all her other faculties.

I hoped it was an isolated incident, though the where, when and why baffled me. Logic dictated that it must have happened at home, when she was on her own. The opportunity to perform this intimate task wouldn't really have presented itself outside, because she never went anywhere by herself now. It remained a mystery for a few weeks.

***

Towards the end of April, the day centre contacted me to say that, with regret, they felt that Joan was no longer benefitting from the time spent there. Panic gripped me. This was a disaster. I went in search of Trish at the memory clinic. She was pragmatic about it all. In her calm, authoritative voice, she told me that Joan's inability to cope with the day centre marked the start of a new chapter headed Residential Care.

'She's not ready for that,' I said.

I was defensive, seeing this statement as a reproach on my ability to care for my mother at home. Trish leant back in her chair and waited for me to suppress the rising panic enough to hear her out.

'Joan is ready, but you're not. You can't deny that you're finding it difficult to keep all the balls up in the air. You have to plan ahead before the crisis comes, while you and Joan still have choices.'

Trish's words were firm, an anchor in my teetering world.

'We'll arrange for Joan to come into the clinic for respite care and during that time we'll do a proper assessment and take it from there. We can move as slowly as you want to, but we have to plan the next stage together.'

The wheels were set in motion, and my mother, tense and tearful with apprehension, went into the clinic for one week. I visited every day, except for the day that she was brought back home, to assess how well (or not) she coped with daily activities.

I was also interviewed to ascertain how much care I had to provide to assist Joan to live on her own. The panel of experts seated before me consisted of the consultant geriatrician (the Greek god), Trish from the memory clinic and an occupational therapist. They proceeded to interrogate me.

'Is your mum able to dress herself, because she seems unable to do so in the clinic?'

'Well, no,' I replied, 'I have to dress and undress her and supervise her shower.'

'Can Joan cook or prepare a meal for herself?'

'No. I provide all her meals now.'

'How about at night, is she safe to be left alone do you think?'

'Not entirely. I have to lock her in and then I hide behind a parked car and wait. Mum takes a while to settle. She will repeatedly come to try the door, presumably to check that it's been locked. I'm afraid that if she works out how to unlock it, she'll wander off into the night looking for me. Of course, if there was a fire, Mum wouldn't be able to get out, simply because she can't figure out how to lock or unlock the door anymore. She also has to have a light on in her bedroom all night, but even so, if she wakes, she has no idea where she is.'

I briefly mentioned that my mother now had a commode in her bedroom, because she was unable to locate the bathroom at night. During the day this didn't appear to pose a problem, but if she woke at night, her brain remained in neutral and didn't appear to kick into any gear. Come the morning, I had to follow the excrement and urine trails to wherever they lead.

After the poo in the bag incident, which I'd hoped, for some unlikely and desperate reason, was an isolated occurrence, losing the toilet had become a regular event. I'd find urine soaked nightdresses screwed up in the back of cupboards and drawers and little packages of excrement, neatly wrapped and hidden away. This only happened during the night and seemed more to do with total confusion about the layout of her home, than incontinence.

Installing the commode had reduced the frequency of accidents. I say reduced, because it only worked if Mum got out of bed on the side where the commode had been placed. I suspected that it only worked then, because she couldn't get past the commode, unless she climbed over it.

The panel of experts in dementia nodded sagely and wrote things down on clipboards.

'And how are you coping?' the Greek god asked.

I hadn't expected that question. I wasn't ready to admit that I was so tired, stressed and depressed that I just wanted to go to sleep and never wake up. I didn't want to tell them that I'd never been close to Joan. I found even touching her difficult and repulsive now. I couldn't say that I often shouted at her. I'd always give myself a lecture on loving kindness and understanding before going to see her, but these days, two minutes in her presence, and I was in danger of losing control. I over compensated by keeping her bungalow and garden in pristine condition, a thankless and unnecessary task. I wasn't asked how my marriage was holding up under the strain and for that I was grateful.

'It's difficult...' I said.

The panel consolidated their findings. According to Joan, she was managing just fine at home. Yes, she cooked and cleaned for herself and could work the washing machine, TV, shower, etc. Needless to say her performance, on a trial run at home, didn't match her verbal assurance, but then they knew it wouldn't.

Their assessment was that Joan was ready for residential care. No, she hadn't actually agreed to this, but fear of the unknown would render this unlikely. Joan had admitted, however, that she was anxious being on her own now. With a stab of guilt, I realised that I'd never asked and certainly didn't know that was how she felt. I'd failed her and acknowledgment of this was flooding my cheeks. The panel, as if collectively reading my mind, assured me that they understood that I wasn't ready to let go, they understood that I would feel as if I'd failed. They weren't wrong.

Chapter Seven

They suggested that I choose a residential home that would be suitable. Social Services gave me a list of accredited homes but they weren't permitted to recommend particular ones. I was told that it would be preferable to select a small home, to give Joan the best opportunity of finding her way around. It would also have to be a home that accepted a percentage of elderly mentally ill (EMI) clients as that was now Joan's classification.

The advice was that when I'd found a home, they would arrange for my mother to attend on a day basis, perhaps two days a week, to give me a break, and to acclimatise Joan. Thus the transition from being cared for in her own home to residential care would be as painless as possible.

I came away with a list and a couple of mother-free days to research available homes. I was already familiar with some of the residential homes on the list because I'd worked in them, but I wouldn't be inclined to put my mother there. The standard of care ranged from passable to downright appalling.

I made a few enquiries from people I knew, who were still employed as care workers and took my initial findings to the charge nurse at Abbotsvale. Paul had been appointed as my mother's key worker, an unfortunate choice since her aversion to men had intensified over the last few months. Still, Paul was a likable bloke and always very approachable.

I pushed the list towards him, the homes of preference underlined.

'I know you can't recommend, but can you indicate if I'm way off target here?'

Paul scrutinised the list. Using his pen as a pointer, together with facial expressions and body language, he conveyed the information I required. My list of four was whittled down to two, both of which, if I'd read his mime act right, were deemed to be suitable. I was left with the task of visiting both places to have a look around, and to ascertain if they would be willing to take Mum when a vacancy came up, and on a day basis before that.

I favoured one home over the other by some margin. The one place, isolated from life down a quiet lane, had a manageress who was stacked like a female bodybuilder, and she had an intimidating manner to go with her bulk. The home, though clean and sweet-smelling, was like a rabbit warren. I could see that Mum wouldn't have a hope of learning the layout.

I opted for Mount Kingsley, which has since reverted to a private residence. They advertised their day care facilities, and I was impressed with the thought that had gone into the structure of the activities provided and the freedom of movement given to the residents. It was a large Victorian building, but the ground floor had lounge, kitchen, bedrooms, toilets, door to the garden and staircase to additional bedrooms, all coming from a spacious central reception hall. Outside was a large garden with a small outdoor swimming pool and plenty of seating scattered around.

Having worked in residential care, I knew not to be overly concerned about the décor. Most clients prefer homely to the luxury hotel look. En suite facilities are wasted on people with advanced dementia. A commode in each room and plenty of toilet/bath/shower rooms are all that's required.

A simple layout is good, so that the terminally bewildered have a fighting chance of finding their way around the building. One would expect staff to be friendly to both residents and visitors but that's not necessarily so. Staff that have been trained to deal with the unique requirements of clients with dementia would be excellent, but rare in my experience.

I think it's reasonable to expect that in-house courses are held regularly to teach staff how to care for the elderly. From how to put on an incontinence pad correctly (yes, there is a right and wrong way) to the importance of stimulation, exercise and adequate fluid intake. New, inexperienced staff shouldn't be let loose on residents before all the basic training has been given.

Ideally, residential care should be less about containment and more about enhancement. Are the chairs placed in informal groupings? Does the hairdresser call each week? Can residents be involved in the shopping, gardening, cooking, and even simple maintenance jobs? Is there access to a library with a regular turnover of books? Are there activities on offer that encourage socialisation and stimulate the brain? Is there regular opportunity to venture outside the home, to go for a pint or a cup of coffee, a visit to the cinema or theatre, maybe just a walk in the park? Is in-house entertainment provided?

Not much to ask you'd think, but unfortunately there are still more bad care homes out there than there are good ones and the majority fall somewhere in between.

It's unfortunate that the pay for carers remains inadequate and although relevant NVQs are often an advertised requirement, it's still not universal by any means. If, as an employer, your expectations of your staff are low, reflected by the pay and lack of qualifications and/or training, you will get the staff you deserve. They are not necessarily the staff to best serve your paying customers, whether privately funded or in receipt of local Authority funding.

Mount Kingsley ticked a good many of the boxes, and Mrs Arnold was a larger than life personality. She had a background as a social worker and appeared to run a fairly tight ship. It helped that I had inside information in the form of two friends who already worked there and I trusted their opinion, which was favourable.

The plan was that Mum would come home on the understanding that she would attend Mount Kingsley for two days a week, on a day care basis. When a place became available she would enter full-time residential care. Not that my mother was told about the long term arrangement. Sufficient unto the day…

Mum had to fund the day care herself and her full-time care, when it came, would also be self-funded. If anyone is under the illusion that this means better care, be assured or reassured, depending on your finances, that this isn't always the case. The two worst homes that I've ever worked in were both nursing homes that only took self-funded clients. I resigned from both, simply because I couldn't be party to the deplorable levels of care. They both had a veneer of top class service. Always scratch beneath the surface and try before you buy. Give the home a month's test run before making a commitment.

I had to provide transport to and from Mount Kingsley, but arrival and departure was flexible. This arrangement worked better than the stress of getting Mum ready for the minibus to the day centre. She settled in well, always reluctant to go, but equally reluctant to leave and far more animated after her day spent there. I was optimistic that when Mum moved into full-time care, the transition would be less traumatic than I'd envisaged. That move came out of the blue.

***

Joan now required assistance with all aspects of daily life. She was no longer able to dress herself without considerable help. Left to her own devices she favoured the layered approach to daywear: several pairs of pants, petticoats and bras, upside down, back to front, inside out. But she rarely progressed to covering her underwear. I'd lay her clothes out the night before, but they were ignored as she raided drawers, wardrobe and linen basket in search of alternative attire. Every morning, once Jake had gone off to school, I would hot foot it round to Mum's to rectify the fashion disasters and render her fit for viewing, whether attending Abbotsvale or Mount Kingsley.

Showering was done in the evening because her ability to turn the shower on and off had gone and I had to be in attendance. Some functions were maintained using very simple step by step written instructions, which meant that her bungalow looked like a public notice board. The ability to perform simple tasks, such as turning light switches on and off, disappeared altogether. My mother was unable to relate the switch to the light bulb. This meant I needed to go round in the evening to perform the lighting up ceremony, otherwise she'd remain sitting in the dark, apart from a small side light that operated by a time switch. Yet the relatively complicated mechanism that opened and closed, locked and unlocked her sliding patio door, she was still able to operate, following the prompt sheet stuck to the wall.

Meals had to be provided by me. Mum may still have been able to make a cup of tea and possibly some rudimentary meal, but was not inclined to do so. Whether she no longer registered hunger or thirst, so lacked the incentive to prepare food or make a drink or had simply forgotten how, I wasn't sure. But she always ate the meals that were prepared for her, so I guess it was just another skill on the list headed Departed. I was exhausted and stressed in my role as main care provider for Joan. Up to this point there had been workable, if not ideal, compromises. Now there were too many problems and too few solutions. The final straw always comes when you least expect it.

On that fateful day, I was running late trying to rectify the results of my mother's night time activities and get her ready for Abbotsvale. She'd been gardening, a carer's euphemistic term for fingernails full of excrement. Her nightdress had also been a victim of this nocturnal activity. The nightdress, together with the bathroom mat, which had met a similar fate, were slung into the laundry basket to be dealt with as soon as I'd taken Mum to the centre.

The day passed, other issues cropped up, and I totally forgot to go back to the bungalow. I picked Mum up just after 3.30pm, took her home and made her some tea. I left with the habitual reassurance that I'd be back as soon as I'd fed my family. Some three hours later I returned to settle her for the evening.

'Hi, it's only me.'

No answer. I called again.

'Hi, Mum.'

Out of the spare bedroom, which housed the linen basket, wandered my bewildered mother, wearing the faeces encrusted nightdress over her day clothes, the bath mat having been laid out in front of the spare bed.

I lost it. A statement of fact.

I slammed Joan up against the wall, one hand around her throat and the other hand clenched around her clothing and thrust into her shoulder. I was screaming into her face. I can't remember the words, just the viciousness and anger.

I recall her repeating over and over, 'I'm sorry, I'm sorry, I'll be a good girl, Mummy, I'll be good.'

It's strange to me that the final straw is rarely the biggest or heaviest, it's usually the blade of grass, so light, that in isolation it's insignificant. I was out of control and terrified. Distraught and hysterical, I ran from the scene, desperate to escape from Joan and from myself.

I pounded the pavements until my legs were shaking and threatening to give way with the exertion. My breath was coming in ragged gasps from a chest that felt it was going to split in two. Then the tears came as I slumped, in the darkness, out of sight, against the wall of a block of garages.

I went back, of course, remorseful and apologetic, but in my mind the damage was done. I could have killed her, I didn't, but in that moment I could have. She was in danger, because I could no longer trust myself.

The one and only blessing of dementia is that by the next morning Mum appeared to have forgotten all that had taken place the evening before. I'd spent a sleepless night deciding what to do. It was obvious that I'd reached the edge and was now staring into the abyss at the end of this phase as my mother's carer. I made an emergency appointment with the GP and poured out what had happened and what I feared might happen.

'For her own safety she needs to be in residential care. I obviously can't cope anymore.'

He understood. No recriminations. I'd have felt better if he'd seen fit to tell me what an awful person I was. It was what I deserved. I begged for an increase in my antidepressants, which was granted.

***

Within the week Joan was booked into Abbotsvale, to await transfer into residential care. The doctor had taken me seriously.

Four weeks later, after two meetings with the geriatrician and Trish from Abbotsvale, it was done and dusted. Mrs Arnold had a vacant room at Mount Kingsley. I chose and purchased a pretty, creamy-yellow paint for the walls of Mum's room to cover the bleak blue chosen by the previous occupant. Mr Arnold did the painting, moaning continuously about the smell of the paint.

My mother was tearful at leaving Abbotsvale which, in one month, had become home. Abbotsvale only offered respite care. It was run on similar lines to a hospital so was unsuitable for long term residential care. In any event, we were now at the point of no return.

Being upstairs, the room at Mount Kingsley wasn't ideal. Mum was getting doddery on stairs, but she only had to come down them once a day, in the morning and up again at night, to go to bed, and she'd have an escort. I left my mother at the home, as she began her month's trial in full-time residential care.

For the most part, the first month went well, my mother formed a childlike attachment to Mrs Arnold and often went with her into town to help with the shopping. She also assisted in the kitchen, which was one reason why I rarely ate their homemade cakes.

A friend of mine, Bill, ran an art class there, but my mother didn't appear to be interested in exploring her artistic tendencies. But she did enjoy the armchair keep fit programme using ribbons, the indoor skittles and outings for tea at various homes of participating hosts. They also had a pianist who came in on a regular basis to play all the old, popular songs, hysterically badly, but nobody seemed to mind. I was delighted to see Mum become friends with another elderly lady, called Edith. They would always sit together.

At the end of the trial period, Mrs Arnold, Bob and I had a meeting to discuss Joan's suitability for the home. We needed to provide some sports bras for ease of dressing and proper handkerchiefs. Her habit of shredding tissues was making extra work, clearing the snow drifts that covered her bedroom floor. Beyond that, Joan was pronounced an ideal resident. A permanent place was offered, and we were happy to accept it.

PART 3

Chapter Eight

I didn't anticipate how difficult it would be to get my life back after nearly four years of mother-care. I thought I could just slip back into life as it'd been before. Now I had to find work again, and return to the cold silence of the marital home, without the distraction of looking after Mum.

I got a temporary job, working nights at a local factory. The job was only for two months, packing potpourri for various retail outlets. I enjoyed the work. Being part of a process with a product at the end of it is satisfying, without the stress of responsibility. It filled a gap while I looked for something more permanent. I was sorry when the contract ended. By then I'd secured employment as a cleaner at the home and sports injury clinic run by two doctors, plus a care assistant's post in a home for adults with learning difficulties. Both part-time positions, but together added up to enough to pay my way at home.

The hours I worked left me time to visit my mother, look after my own home, and keep an eye on the bungalow. Bob was all for letting it, but I wanted to hang on for a while, I don't really know why. I suppose I was still using it to escape from the increasingly oppressive atmosphere at home and was reluctant to lose it. Anyway I wanted to sell it and invest the money to fund Mum's care, which wasn't going to come cheap and seemed likely to be long term. Moreover, I didn't want the responsibility of being cast in the role of landlord, which I strongly suspected would fall to me, or the expense of letting it through an agent. I persuaded Bob to leave things as they were for a while.

I'd been worried about whether Mum would settle into her new life, but I was having major problems settling back into my old one. I now had too much time to focus on the sham that was my marriage. It'd been nearly thirteen years since my husband had spoken to me conversationally and twelve years since we'd shared a bed. He went out most evenings, I'd no idea where. I cooked and cleaned, but he'd taken over certain personal tasks. Ray would remove his clothes from the ironing pile and iron them himself, no one else's, just his own. The trousers I would shorten for him when he bought new ones, he now took somewhere else to be altered. I used to cut his hair, now I was forbidden physical contact of any kind. I was struggling with ongoing depression, and I couldn't cope with the situation anymore, I wanted out.

My husband had been seen on several occasions in the company of another woman, Penny, the ex-girlfriend. I'd always suspected he'd been involved with her, on and off, throughout our marriage, but had no proof. I'd clung on this long in the desperate hope that he'd love me, but I had to face the fact that what he wanted was me gone. He was prepared to sit it out and continue the silent torture until he achieved that goal.

I couldn't settle and decided to take a holiday. Family holidays had long since ceased. For several years after Ray stopped communications, I'd insisted on a family holiday each year. It was a bizarre affair. In the beginning we hired a camper van and then a few years in, Ray bought a touring caravan. It was used for the statutory two weeks per annum, then put into storage.

For about eight years we kept up this charade. Minimal contact throughout the year, Ray refusing to speak and refusing to allow me use of the car, except for weekly shopping. The supermarket run was unaccompanied by Ray of course, but timed, just in case I had the audacity to visit a friend en route. I was totally shut out of his social life. Looking back, I can see that I was treated worse than a servant. At the very least, you have to be polite to hired help or they quit. He was never physically abusive, but the emotional and mental abuse were equally as damaging.

Under the circumstances, a miracle took place every year before we reached the first night's destination of this annual event. Ray became transformed into the model husband. It was wonderful. He spoke to me as if I was his much-loved wife, he joked, he laughed and we conversed amicably. He was the man I fell in love with, and every year I would fall in love with him all over again. As soon as we returned and stepped over the threshold of our home, the shutters came down. I was persona non grata once more.

The annual family holiday stopped when Jake began secondary education. By then he'd became more aware that his parents' relationship wasn't normal. He was no longer inclined towards family holidays with his weird parents, and I have to admit I was grateful for that.

I booked a week in Tunisia. I'd never been on a plane, had never been abroad, didn't even own a passport, so getting one was my first step.

I don't know why I did it or even how. I blame the Paroxetine. A side effect of this particular antidepressant, later recognised and utilised by the pharmaceutical company, was a reduction in inhibitions and shyness. I can only think I was cashing in on this anomaly, I certainly can't imagine doing it now. I left a note on the fridge, with the hotel's details.

'Gone to Tunisia for a week, meals are in the freezer.'

My son later told me that his father was astounded to the point of getting the atlas out to discover where Tunisia actually was. His astonishment turned to apoplexy when he realised that Tunisia was in Africa. I think Jake was quite impressed by his mother's spirit of adventure. When I phoned him during the week, from a phone shop in the centre of Sousse, I got the impression that I'd earned some kudos. That, from a sixteen-year-old, is hard to come by.

I loved Tunisia. It was a package holiday so quite safe as long as you took the advice of the tour guide. There were so many "firsts" for me, it was amazingly liberating and confidence building. I was middle-aged and overweight, but it was of no consequence. I joined up with two other single, middle-aged women who, being veterans of the package holiday scene, happily took me under their wing. We did all the touristy things, the Arabian night out, the camel ride into the Sahara to watch the sunset, still in my top ten of experiences that I'll never forget.

I was asked out for a drink by the head waiter a couple of days after he'd retrieved me from the German restaurant on my first night.

Apparently, it was the Tunisians' perception that Germans and British didn't get on, therefore they needed to have separate restaurants to minimise bloodshed. I'd strayed into the wrong place, oblivious to the fact that I didn't belong there. I have no idea in what way I stood out as not being German, but somebody must have shopped me to the maitre d' and I was removed. An international incident averted.

Unfortunately, the Tunisians' understanding of what the British like to eat did make me wish, at times, that I was German. Their food had looked vastly more interesting than the fare in our restaurant. Did the Brits still eat pink blancmange? I didn't take the head waiter up on his offer but he'd no idea what his invitation did for my self esteem. The fact that he continued to be very attentive throughout that week was wonderful. I wished I could have bottled that euphoric sensation and brought it home with me.

On my last night, ensconced on my balcony, I listened to the cacophony of sparrows as they squabbled over roosting pitches in the trees below. I wept at the thought of going home. I'd had a week of social wellbeing, others had wanted to include me in their company. I wasn't that worthless person my husband wanted me to believe I'd become.

'Not a day goes by when you're not an inconvenience to me,' he'd said. 'Nobody comes to visit us because of you.'

Ray had thrown these phrases at me, always said as a controlled statement, for maximum impact.

I couldn't continue like this, something had to change.

As I could have predicted, there was no response from my husband on my return. It was as if he'd never noticed I'd been away. He wouldn't acknowledge my homecoming for good or for bad. It was the final straw.

The holiday had heightened my sense of grieving for the relationship with Ray that I wanted so badly. I'd reached the end of my endurance. Emotionally and mentally, I was losing control. The drug-induced protective bubble wrap was fast being popped, bubble by bubble.

***

Early in the Spring of 1998, I booked an appointment with a solicitor to talk through my survival plan. Jake was old enough to know what was going on. Much later it would become plain that he knew a lot more than I'd given him credit for, but didn't know how, or even if, he should tell me. He accepted the status quo because the situation at home had always been the same, he knew nothing different. But he admitted that it was an uncomfortable place to be and quite unlike the homes of his close friends, whose parents had marriages that were all rock solid.

I explained to the solicitor that I couldn't have a divorce because my faith only recognised divorce on the grounds of adultery and although I had reason to believe that adultery had taken place, I couldn't prove it. A judicial separation was the way forward. This ensured that all the finances and where Jake would live, would be sorted out legally, but as a couple we'd still be married. I then dropped the bombshell that I just wanted half the value of the house and whatever bits of furniture I needed to take with me (which wouldn't be much). The solicitor, having ascertained Ray's occupation, plus a guesstimate at his pension prospects, became very animated.

'You're entitled to so much more and a share of your husband's pension,' he told me. 'Whatever you decide now will be legally binding, even if you divorce later. You must think this through carefully.'

I had thought it through, I'd done little else for weeks, but I couldn't explain that I was bone weary and just wanted to escape. I had to make this as easy and palatable as possible. I no longer had the strength to fight the legal battle that I knew would ensue if I wanted disclosure of earnings, savings and pension entitlements. I'd never been told what Ray's income was, we had no shared bank account and documentation about everything was kept elsewhere, certainly not in the house. He handed over housekeeping money, in cash, at the end of each month. That, together with my earnings, was all I was to expect to cover the list of regular outgoings that were deemed to be my responsibility.

I stood my ground. The solicitor wouldn't act on my behalf until I'd signed a disclaimer to say that I'd gone against his express recommendation and advice.

Understandable from his point of view. I signed. First hurdle over.

Informing Ray was the next hurdle. Did I want the solicitor to write to him or would I tell him myself? Having worked for a firm of solicitors for a brief while I'd seen, first hand, how they manage to cause contention where there was none to start with. I didn't want to risk making matters worse, but neither did I relish the idea of making our judicial separation the subject of an alien concept in our relationship, a face to face discussion.

My guess was that he would be jubilant that I'd finally caved in and was going, but he would be far from delighted that I wanted half of the property. I was convinced that he'd hoped I'd just go and leave him with it all. I'm sure that's what he'd been waiting for, all these years. I was heartened by the solicitor's words, intoned morosely because he was unable to do what, in his opinion, was his best for me.

'He'll never get an offer as good as this. If I was in his shoes, I'd bite your hand off up to the elbow before you come to your senses and change your mind.'

I decided to write to Ray, outlining what I intended to do and asking him to get himself a solicitor so that they could sort out the details. Before I wrote to Ray, I had to tell Jake. That was the hardest thing I'd ever done. How was this going to affect him and how was it going to affect our relationship? I was in danger of appearing to be the bad guy here. After all, I was the one who was bailing out.

Although sad that the parting of ways was becoming reality, Jake was remarkably calm and stoical about it all, but said that he wanted to come with me. I'd already thought this through. Although I dearly wanted him to live with me, my fear was that his father would see it as an act of treachery on Jake's part and sever the already fragile relationship that existed between them. I explained my fears to my son. Thankfully, he understood my reasoning and didn't dispute that this could be the outcome, if he chose to join me.

At least this way, Jake would have an opportunity to develop a meaningful relationship with his father, without the elephant in the room — me. Jake had assumed the role of diplomat over the years, trying hard to please both parents while drawing further away, as is the default position with teenagers under the best of circumstances. Anyway, at that moment, I'd no idea where I was going.

I agonised over the letter for days. Not about whether I would go through with it or not, my mind was made up, but how to word it. I ended up with a matter of fact, business-like directive:

Why, in precise terms, I was writing rather than talking.

Why I couldn't offer him a divorce at this particular time.

What I wanted.

What I would give.

What I didn't want.

The rider.

This was that Jake would have the freedom, without pressure or persecution, to visit, stay or live with me, if and whenever he wished to, and if either of us wanted to file for divorce at anytime in the future, Ray was to agree to bear the total cost of the proceedings.

It was done and I handed it to Ray, wordlessly. I notified my solicitor and enclosed a copy of the letter. Now I had to wait.

My timing of events was dire as it turned out, because the following night Ray's brother died unexpectedly from a heart attack. I wished I could have turned back time and the letter had never existed, but the worst of it was that I'd no idea how Ray felt about our impending separation or his brother's death. How do you live with somebody for so many years and have no clue what's in their heart or head?

I shelved things for a few weeks and heard nothing from Ray, not a flicker, not an indicator that he'd acted on the letter or even read it. His life seemed to have returned to normal after the funeral and inevitable aftermath. How long was long enough to wait for a response? I'd no idea. I confronted him.

'This offer is only open for a limited time, I've been advised that I'm entitled to a lot more. At the moment I'm going against my solicitor's advice just to make this easy, but if I don't hear from you very soon, I'll withdraw this offer and allow the solicitor to do things his way.'

I got the sentence out in one breath, my heart pounding in my throat. Ray looked at me and maintained the level voice of barely suppressed disdain.

'My solicitor has already written to yours to agree to your conditions. Satisfied?'

Strangely enough, no. There was this overwhelming desire in me to break this façade of indifference. Inside I ached and hurt, I wanted him to care but he didn't, I wanted him to shout and scream at me but he wouldn't and I'd now cut the cord and felt as if I was drifting into the whirlpool.

Chapter Nine

My judicial separation was going through, albeit slowly. I had to make plans. To the onlooker, nothing had changed at home. I intended to stay until Jake had completed his GCSEs, so my estimated date of departure was June.

I knew what capital I had to work with now our house had been valued. I'd need full-time work to keep me solvent and somewhere to live. Tension in the house had lessened, I guess because Ray had achieved his goal. He was still maintaining the silent treatment, but the parting of the ways was in sight. To me, the atmosphere felt less toxic.

My mother had regressed to her boarding school days and had developed a schoolgirl crush on Mrs Arnold, but her mental deterioration was relentless. Her speech was now virtually unintelligible. It wasn't just that the words didn't form a coherent sentence, but her ability to form words at all had all but disappeared. Mum had also become paranoid and her dislike of men was now entrenched. Apart from Edith, Mrs Arnold, Bob and me, she wasn't too enamoured with people in general and was becoming a clinging vine to the chosen few.

The exception to this embargo was my mother's youngest sister, Barbara, who came down from Birmingham a couple of times during Mum's first year in residential care. Barbara was a gregarious personality, and her broad Birmingham accent may have reminded Mum of her childhood. Whether she recognised Barbara as her sister or not, Mum beamed a radiant smile in her direction and all her outward tension melted for a while.

One night, my mother's friend, Edith, became ill and was calling out for help. In small residential homes at that time, as long as someone adequately qualified was on the premises at night, the rules didn't require waking care staff to be on duty. The Arnolds were asleep upstairs in their flat. Edith's bedroom was on the ground floor, and Edith, for whatever reason, couldn't ring her call bell, so they didn't hear her. From her room upstairs, my mother heard her friend's cry for assistance. She navigated her way downstairs to Edith's room and sat with her, murmuring incoherently and patting Edith's hand. Somewhere in her brain, she must have reasoned that this wasn't enough and went in search of help.

Back upstairs she found the door to Mr and Mrs Arnold's flat and banged on it, until she woke them. I don't know who was more surprised, the Arnolds, at seeing Joan at the door to their private quarters, or me, when the story was retold.

After a short spell in hospital, Edith made a full recovery. Joan was taken to visit her. Extra staff were employed for night duty, and a new resident, an elderly gentleman, joined the happy throng.

The new addition to Mount Kingsley, Jim, took a shine to Edith, and a relationship blossomed. Jim and Edith wanted to sit together in the lounge and at mealtimes. My mother was shut out of this cosy twosome. I think, had she been more amenable towards men, it may not have evolved in that way. I'm sure Jim would've been quite happy to have developed his harem. As it was, Mum's hatred of men and Jim, in particular, stepped up a notch or three. Although most of my mother's meaningful language had deserted her and the words she was left with, made little sense, her thoughts about Jim were crystal clear. The verbal description was unintelligible, but the venom, with which she spat out her condemnation, every time she saw him, was scary. Jim was totally oblivious to all this, but then he only had eyes for Edith.

***

My brother made little comment about my proposed marital separation from Ray. It was a difficult situation for him. Bob only knew Ray as a drinking buddy, the guy at the bar with the acerbic sense of humour, usually at someone else's expense. Ray knew how to run a pub and had been invaluable to Bob and his business partner when they embarked on their own pub and restaurant business. Bob's loyalties were divided. Although he didn't want to be taking sides, by his silence on the subject and his continued friendship with Ray, he did.

Bob knew from my parents what the atmosphere was like in our house. Ray didn't behave any differently towards me just because my parents were there. That was the reason they'd chosen to stay with my brother for the last few years of visits to Devon.

At the time, I'd felt devalued by them, both for myself and for my son who would've liked his grandparents staying with us. I was crushed that knowing the situation, they couldn't see fit to support us by dividing their holiday between my brother and me. By their decision, they displayed a perverse acceptance of Ray's behaviour. But perhaps my mother's early onset of dementia was too stressful for my father to handle, within the hostile environment of my home.

Still, I'd made my choice to go it alone. I had, to all intents and purposes, been alone for the last thirteen years, but now I was taking sole responsibility for the rest of my life. Where to start?

I needed somewhere to live. The estate agent gave me the details of two small cottages on the other side of the River Torridge, known on the map as East-the-Water, or Shamwickshire to the locals, but still in Bideford. I discounted one because it had no garden at all or anywhere to park the ancient Ford Fiesta.

The other cottage needed renovating. There was no kitchen, just a sink and draining board, no heating or double glazing and the back roof required some serious attention, but it was basically sound. It was a small, two up two down, terraced cottage, with a lean-to kitchen, a tiny courtyard garden and a shed, which would've once housed the toilet. The bathroom was downstairs, sited where the original kitchen would've been. It cried out for some serious TLC, a kindred spirit. On the practical side its need for modernisation was reflected in the cheap price tag.

Bob suggested that I borrow the money from Mum's account, until I received my half of the marital home and so I bought it. Any spare time I had was spent there, wielding a paintbrush, while dreaming and planning what I would do to make this little cottage into my home.

My brother agreed to sell the bungalow. I wasn't going to be around to keep an eye on it, and Mum was as settled at Mount Kingsley as she was ever going to be. I couldn't imagine a situation where my mother would be returning home. The son and daughter-in-law of the couple next door still wanted it. We sold it to them for the amount Mum had paid for the bungalow. They were delighted, and we cut out the expense of an estate agent.

**

Letters drifted to and fro between solicitors and Jake was in the middle of GCSE exams. At Mount Kingsley, Mum was enjoying the warm weather of late spring. She'd developed a raw rash on her face, which wouldn't heal. After some discussion with the care staff and several attempts with various creams, I remembered that Mum had once told me that she never used soap on her face. The staff stopped the use of soap and the rash disappeared. I was left wondering if she had, in some way, tried to communicate her allergic reaction to soap, but was unable to make herself understood. I felt guilty for being too preoccupied with other matters to recall this isolated, but important detail of an obscure conversation that took place years ago.

I took Mum to see my cottage, confident that any secrets would be safe with her. I tried to explain about my impending separation and that I'd be moving into my new home soon. I'd no idea how much she understood, but suddenly she was grabbing my hand and pulling me towards the front door and out into the street. There seemed a frantic need to get back to Mount Kingsley, so we returned, at breakneck speed.

The staff whisked her away as soon as she entered the building, only to return to reassure me that my mother had just needed the toilet. She was, they said, beginning to have the occasional accident, which upset her so much they were thinking about providing incontinence pads for her now. My heart sank. Joan had now entered my area of expertise, she'd crept over the line into nursing care, rather than residential care. It had happened so quickly, in less than twelve months.

Some residential homes won't permit clients to remain with them if they become incontinent, as they're often ill-equipped and without sufficient staff to deal with the increase in workload that comes with regular toileting and changing. Mrs Arnold assured me that they had it covered and were quite happy to keep Joan with them.

'This is her home,' she said.

That was reassuring, but nevertheless, I left there with a heavy heart at the thought of my mother being reduced to this pathetic figure. A bewildered woman, whose world was shrinking by the week, no longer able to communicate her needs adequately and now having to suffer the indignity of being unable to control her own bladder.

With the bungalow sold, I was using the cottage as my place of peace and security and had already started to undertake the work I was able to do myself. As there wasn't one straight or even wall in the place, I stripped off the loose plaster and slapped a textured finish on the lot. I was quite conservative in the lounge, applying a stippled effect to undergo this transformation. I got more adventurous as I moved through the house. I covered the landing and stairwell in overlapping swirls that probably still remain as a testimony to my retro artistic endeavours, as it would be a daunting task to remove.

I ripped out the boards fixed over the fireplace in the lounge and uncovered an original Victorian cast iron fireplace, showing its age, but nothing that elbow grease and paint couldn't put right. It was an extravagance, but I had the chimney swept and a custom built gas fire, with fake coal and flame effect, fitted into the grate. I purchased a bed, settee, pine table and chairs and scrounged a cooker from a friend who had one going spare. Everything else was coming from the marital home, salvaged from the bungalow, or would be built in at a later date.

Back in February, June seemed an eternity away, but now the time had come. The day I was to move out of the marital home had arrived. While Ray was at work, I stashed all the bits and pieces that I considered mine, the contents of the box room that had served as my bedroom for the last twelve years.

This included my pet rat, Roxy. She'd been bought by me for Jake, but without prior consent from Ray, which meant Jake wasn't permitted to keep it. I adopted Roxy, and she lived in my box room. When I'd visited Mum in her bungalow, Roxy would often travel on my shoulder, hidden under my hood out of sight, if Ray was about. Mum was fascinated by her and didn't seem at all appalled at having a rat in her home.

Seeing Roxy disappear into the back of the Fiesta, Jake became concerned about our cat.

'Dad kicks it when you're not around, did you know that?'

I didn't, but I wasn't surprised.

Jake had wanted a dog when he was about nine years old. As he was an only child, I thought it was a good idea. Ray had refused to even think about it, but reluctantly permitted a cat. Not quite the same impetus, but Jake's first kitten was an instant success.

Gizmo was an endearing and adventurous silver tabby, too adventurous as it turned out. At five months old, he escaped out of the house, ran into the road and went straight under the wheels of a moving car. Jake was inconsolable, Gizmo had been an exceptionally charismatic cat.

I let a few weeks pass and then decided to get another kitten. Jake and I went to a local cat rescue centre to choose one. My son carefully considered the enclosure full of kittens of every colour that kittens come in. He chose a black one with white toes and perfect Felix facial markings.

'Why that one?' I said.

'Because she's so different from Gizmo,' Jake replied. 'All the others ran towards us and are playing together, but this one ran away from us and doesn't want to be with the others. I don't think that she'll be as adventurous as Gizmo, but that's good, because it'll keep her safe.'

I was intrigued and quite impressed by his reasoning and although I understood where he was coming from, I wasn't sure it was the best basis for choosing a pet. Still, Missy (Mistletoe) had been with us for seven years and had proved to be as reclusive and antisocial as had been predicted.

Jake asked if I would take Missy with me. He wasn't around much at this point. At sixteen, he had his own life which, for obvious reasons, wasn't centred around his home. The cat carrier, dishes and food were stashed into the Ford Fiesta which was beginning to bulge at the sides. I just hoped Missy didn't do a disappearing act on me when it was time to leave.

The end of the afternoon came, and Ray was due back from work. Jake was looking apprehensive, and I was trying hard to keep it together, waiting for Ray to come home. I wanted to hand him my contact details, so there would be no dispute as to whether he'd received them or not.

Jake bailed out, before Ray turned up, with the promise that he'd be over to see me as soon as possible. We hugged, I could feel him shaking, or was it me? I went upstairs to check that I'd left nothing behind. While I was up there, Ray returned, came upstairs to his bedroom to get changed out of his office clothes and went back downstairs to watch the news. I returned to the lounge and flitted past him to retrieve the cat from the kitchen and put her into the car. Not a flicker. I retraced my steps into the lounge, with the envelope containing my telephone number and address and stood for a few seconds to the side of him, my arm outstretched. Ray remained cast in stone. I placed the envelope on the settee beside him.

'This is my new address and telephone number,' I said. 'Just in case you need to contact me, which you might, especially if it's something that affects Jake.'

Nothing. No eye contact. No words. He turned his head slightly to acknowledge the envelope beside him and with a slight shrug of one shoulder, he returned to the screen.

With every limb convulsed with tremors and aware of neighbouring net curtains twitching, I left. I drove over to the cottage, removed cat and rat from the car into the kitchen. Then I collapsed onto the stairs and wept and howled with pain, grief, fear and relief, until the gloom of dusk brought its own calm. Under cover of encroaching night, I emptied the car of the remains of my marriage.

***

Coming into September, 1998, I was juggling three part-time jobs, having taken on additional work as a cleaner at a health centre. I'd had the roof of the cottage repaired and a kitchen and large wardrobe fitted. The decorating was my ongoing project on temporary hold while the plumber began to install central heating.

My workload, visiting my mother, plus the activity surrounding the cottage meant I didn't have much time to think, never mind mope. I had a friend with a young daughter living a couple of doors down from me and an older couple, who were proving to be my mainstay, living just up the road. Jake was calling in on a frequent basis, having friends in that part of town. He still found the atmosphere at home heavy going. I had no premonition at all of the next glitch to come.

***

Most days, I was getting home around lunchtime, having started work at 6am. This particular day, I was greeted by the plumber drilling his way to somewhere, from the cupboard under the stairs. He emerged with the announcement that he'd managed to stroke Missy. He was making it a life's goal to make friends with her before he finished this job. She'd made herself scarce throughout all the work that was being done, disappearing to the shed during bad weather or the bottom of the garden, where the sun hit the wall. Before disappearing into the cupboard again, the plumber said.

'By the way, you've got a message from a Mrs Arnold on your answer machine, it sounded urgent.'

I wasn't overly anxious. I often got calls asking me to bring in something for my mother and I was due to visit that afternoon. I rang back. Mrs Arnold wasn't there, but the care worker was unusually insistent that I came in at around 3pm, when Mrs Arnold would be back. She wouldn't say anymore, and I felt no reason to press her, except to ask if Mum was alright. Yes, she assured me, she was.

When I arrived later, Mrs Arnold met me in the car park, an unprecedented greeting, which made me feel uneasy. She asked me to come into a small side lounge that doubled as a staff room. Mrs Arnold was being unusually businesslike, not unfriendly exactly, but unsmiling. Then she dropped the bombshell.

'I regret this very much, but I'm afraid I must ask you to find alternative accommodation for Joan.'

The sentence hung in the air like the sword of Damocles.

'I'm afraid your mother's experiencing an elevated state of anxiety and paranoia and as a result is lashing out at staff and other residents.'

The silence stood between us. I hadn't been aware that I was holding my breath, until the pain in my chest reminded me to breathe. I didn't want to hear anymore.

'A few nights ago, Joan attacked a member of the night staff, breaking her glasses and damaging her face,' Mrs Arnold continued. 'We thought, we hoped, it was an isolated incident, but yesterday afternoon I walked into the lounge, having heard Jim shouting, just in time to prevent Joan using a walking stick to attack a resident. She'd dragged poor little Winnie out of her chair and onto the floor. Joan was standing over her with Winnie's stick in her hands, raised, as if she was about to strike Winnie with it.'

I'm sure my mouth had dropped open at this point. My mother? The paranoia had got worse, but physical violence? Could this really be true? Perhaps it was a cruel joke or mistaken identity. Mrs Arnold could probably read the conflicting thoughts flooding my brain. She expressed sorrow at having to make this decision, but she couldn't put other residents or staff at risk. She spoke in a soft tone, aware that this was hard for me to hear.

'Joan is now at a stage where specialised care has become necessary, Social Services have been informed. As soon as a bed becomes available, Joan will be admitted to Abbotsvale for re-assessment, in a couple of days at the most.'

There was no point protesting, it was a *fait accompli*. I just couldn't grasp that my mother could be responsible for this seemingly unprovoked violence. Mrs Arnold assured me that they would pack up her things and deal with the transfer to Abbotsvale. They would also store her bits of furniture for me, until her final destination had been decided upon. It was the least they could do under the circumstances, she said.

I didn't stay to see Joan. I needed distance between me, Mount Kingsley and my mother.

That evening, I broke the news to Bob. He was baffled and angry in equal measure, but then neither of us had seen this coming, although I felt I should have. Could I have done something to prevent this situation? Mum had been at Mount Kingsley for eleven months. As far as I'd been aware, she felt settled and secure. I knew she'd become very anti-men, but these attacks were on women, one of whom was a little old lady, who never moved from her chair unaided and seldom spoke. Why?

I didn't receive an explanation, not that it would have furnished my mother with a stay of execution. Abbotsvale couldn't shed much light on my mother's behaviour, just to say that it was a common development of Alzheimer's disease.

Nobody appears to have done much research as to why some dementia patients remain passive and others become aggressive, as the illness progresses. I'd come across this unprovoked violence in clients with dementia before. Regrettably, I'd never questioned it, just presumed it was a character trait that had always been present, but was now not able to be controlled.

The other question gnawing at my brain was why I'd never been on the receiving end of my mother's violent outbursts, or even witnessed her in action? I couldn't even recall her smacking me when I was a child, though she may have reasoned that her husband more than compensated for her reluctance to administer corporal punishment. The only time I could recall a violent encounter with my mother, I was the provocateur. A real cat fight, with Joan on the defensive against her fifteen-year-old daughter. I came away with a handful of her hair, which frightened me as much as it must have hurt her.

***

Abbotsvale decided that Joan was no longer a suitable candidate for a residential home. She was in need of specialised care in a nursing home for the EMI. In our region, there were only two such places within a reasonable travelling distance. I visited both and hated both. The first one was a rabbit warren and stank of urine. All the rooms were unwelcoming and the décor, politely put, was tired, plus there were no en suite facilities.

I was well aware that an en suite toilet was an unnecessary luxury for advanced dementia patients and indeed that was what I was told by the member of staff showing me around. I knew it, but I didn't want to hear it from this hard-faced woman who was exhibiting thinly-disguised impatience and lacking anything that resembled compassion. I ruled it out. That left me with one.

By the end of that week, the plumber had finished installing central heating and left. Towards the evening, I realised that Missy had gone too. I searched house, garden and street, calling her name. Nothing.

The next day, I left posters on lamp posts and through neighbouring letter boxes. I informed the vet and rang Jake to tell him to be on the lookout, in case she should try to make her way back to her roots. I then curled up in the chair and blubbed noisily. Life seemed grossly unfair.

PART 4

Chapter Ten

The other home was an impressive manor house, Huesneath Moor, situated in an elevated position, overlooking moorland. A fantastic view, as equally wasted on the dementia sufferer as the en suite facilities. The owner, who showed me round, was welcoming and down to earth, with a sense of humour I could relate to and on that particular day the air smelt sweet. Mrs B and her husband owned and ran the home.

Mrs B was a state registered nurse and appeared to know her stuff. She didn't like the unnecessary use of drugs as a medical cosh, a sentiment that I fully endorsed, in theory. I didn't really know enough about use of medication and dementia sufferers to express an informed opinion about how not using medication worked in practice.

Within the home, there was certainly oodles of space for the restless to wander. There were long wide corridors and tucked away seating areas. I did fleetingly wonder how the staff rounded up the residents for meals. Perhaps I should have asked these questions as they flitted through my head, but then, this was it. There was nowhere else.

There was a room vacant, next to the main lounge, a large room with a lovely view and an en suite toilet. Bob had left it up to me, so there was no need and no point in discussing it further. I said yes.

Within two weeks of Joan's eviction from Mount Kingsley, we were on the move to the nursing home for the EMI. Bob and his mate Bill moved Mum's bits of furniture into her room, closely followed by Joan. This time there was no easing her gently into her new home.

My mother was distraught. She wept like a child as I prepared to leave.

'Mum! Mum!' She cried.

Her arms outstretched towards me, her face a mask of fear and total bewilderment.

The nurse on duty took me to one side.

'I suggest that you leave it a few days before you visit,' she said. 'Give Joan time to settle and transfer her dependency onto the staff. We're here for both of you, don't forget that.'

They were reassuring words, genuinely spoken, but I left with a lead weight in my chest.

***

Overnight, my mother went from being a woman with dementia, but secure in the relationships she had and seemingly content, into a frail old lady, who was floundering in this vast cavern of a place. She spent her days wandering aimlessly up and down the corridors, mute, miserable and lost. It broke my heart every time I visited during those first two months.

It wasn't that Mrs B and the staff didn't care, I'm sure that they did. There was music, care assistants painted varnish on nails and chatted to the residents. All the activities that I expected to see. I couldn't put my finger on it exactly, but concluded that Huesneath Moor wasn't a home, it was an institution. Too big, too impersonal. The furniture was functional, chairs chosen, not for comfort, but for ease of getting people into and out of them, with cushions designed to be urinated on. There were no residents helping in the kitchen. I don't recall ever seeing the kitchen. No visits to the shops or the local café, and no pottering about in the garden even though the grounds were vast.

So much more could have been done to extend the range of experiences, but it wasn't. Maybe it was due to lack of imagination, or money. Perhaps it was acceptance of the inevitable fact that the world of the dementia sufferer closes inwards, until any diversion from the norm induces anxiety, reluctance and resistance. But, if these enhanced features were a constant part of everyday life, would that still be the case? I didn't know. The fact remained that the residents were benignly incarcerated within the walls of this manor house.

The other disturbing factor was that, because it was a home designated for the EMI, not all the residents had dementia, some had other forms of mental illness. Other residents had severe learning difficulties, who'd perhaps been cared for by relatives all their lives until this was no longer possible, or had been institutionalised since birth.

There were too many different client groups, each group having their own special needs, never mind the individual requirements of each resident. It didn't work, it was harking back to the huge mental hospitals, long since disbanded, where mentally ill, mentally subnormal (as the terminology was then) and dementia patients were all lumped together under the same roof. Different wards, maybe, but more or less treated the same. I thought those days had gone, but here they were, revisited, under the banner of the Elderly Mentally Ill.

Visiting wasn't easy, with my work schedule. It was a forty minute drive to the home and with encroaching winter, I didn't relish driving through country lanes in the dark. A job was advertised in the local paper for a night care assistant at a local residential and respite home for adults with severe learning difficulties. Four nights of ten-hour shifts and four days off meant consolidated work hours, plus an increased income. The shifts began at 10pm so I could still keep all the fixed aspects of my life intact. On paper it was a no brainer. I applied and got the job after an interview in which I didn't shine, as I was told later by my manager, but my work history (I'd done similar night work before) got me through.

The new job wasn't plain sailing. Most of the night staff had been there for many years and for the most part that wasn't a problem. I was quite happy to dovetail into their way of doing things, they were a good bunch. But I inadvertently crossed swords with one particular member of staff who proceeded to surround herself with an impenetrable wall of silence for an entire ten-hour shift.

Having suffered the silent treatment for thirteen years, I wasn't prepared to endure it again, especially as, again, I'd no idea what I was supposed to have done or not done, so I asked.

Apparently, word had filtered back to this particular member of staff, that in a general conversation with another care worker, I'd expressed surprise that staff were permitted to smoke in rooms shared by the residents. I didn't recall the incident, but it was a cause I'd have been likely to champion. All I could do was state my anti-smoking policy. It wasn't a personal attack, merely an observation that there should, in this enlightened age, be regulations safeguarding the physical health of vulnerable people, who had no actual say in the matter themselves.

This explanation didn't win me an award for diplomacy. Relations remained strained, until a rule was implemented by management, making all residential areas a "no smoking zone" for staff. Anyone needing a nicotine fix had to go outside for it. With that bone of contention removed, animosity ceased overnight and the work environment became tranquil and smoke free.

**

It was November 1998 and life was dropping into a more predictable routine. I managed to get a week's holiday. I had to twist the arm of my friend, Margaret, to persuade her to come with me to Malta. A true Devonshire girl, she didn't much care for holidays and certainly not holidays abroad, but she needed to escape the demands on her time as much as I did, so I nagged her into it. The weather in Malta could have been kinder, but we walked a lot, slept a lot, read a lot and went sightseeing. We lapped up the time that was ours and not in demand by anyone else. The consensus was that a week wasn't long enough.

My visit to my mother, the day after I got back from Malta, was a wake up call. Her teeth had gone missing. How could that possibly happen? Apparently, she had started taking them out as a regular activity, but they'd always been located by staff, usually stuffed down the side of a chair. Now they'd disappeared, despite a vigorous search. There was no way Mum could cooperate sufficiently to enable her to be fitted for a new set of teeth. Management had come to the decision that she would have to manage without them, which allegedly she was already doing, as long as her food was cut up or mashed. It was a done deal. I didn't feel I had much choice but to acquiesce.

My toothless mother was wandering aimlessly, giving no indication that she had any idea at all who I was, after only ten days absence. I didn't think this inevitable regression would upset me as much as it did. Okay, I hadn't been "Jill" for many months, I was usually "Mum" if she referred to me by a name at all. Now there was no glimmer of recognition whatsoever.

I sat in her chair in the corner of the lounge and watched her wandering around the room, up and down the corridor, stopping here and there to touch door handles and objects on tables. In her own world, wherever that was.

'Is it my imagination, or is my mother not as steady on her feet today?' I threw the question out to the nearby staff.

It had already been noted. It transpired that she would now, mid-amble, lie down on the floor.

'Not fall down,' they were quick to assure me. 'Joan will just put herself on the floor.'

Well, I thought, perhaps she's simply worn out. She must cover some miles with this endless wandering.

I was ruminating on this latest evidence of my mother's decline as I watched Joan meander back into the lounge and navigate her way between armchairs which were placed in informal groups throughout the room. Joan wandered up behind the chair where Enid habitually sat. Enid spent her days sleeping, complaining about her aches and pains and knitting, in rotation. With no warning or provocation, Joan grabbed two handfuls of Enid's hair and yanked with all the viciousness of a pub brawl, gums gritted and fists clenched.

When Enid screamed, there was this split second when all onlookers were stunned into paralysis. Suddenly everyone, as a body, sprung into action, shouting at Joan to let go, while trying to prise her hands open. She did let go, more precisely the hair let go, as it parted company with Enid's scalp. Mayhem ensued. Enid was screaming and crying at top volume, inevitably provoking a response from everyone else in the room, residents and staff alike. The only person who remained calm was my mother, who, having released this valve of destructive energy, was serene and compliant. Now, I'd witnessed first hand the reason my mother was here and not at Mount Kingsley.

After the storm, came the post-assault analysis. Members of the staff were now eager to inform me that the honeymoon period had ended, and Joan had been displaying levels of aggression towards them for some weeks. While the carers were trying to assist her with dressing and general care, she would grab at them, digging her fingernails into flesh, yanking at their hair and biting. She hadn't, up to this point, launched an attack on another resident, nor had she shown any aggression towards me or my brother. My heart sank, though my brain flagged up the thought, *I wonder if her teeth went missing by accident or design?*

I reproached myself for such an uncharitable thought and filed it away. I was also beginning to question the wisdom of Mrs B's conviction that the use of medication should be kept to the absolute minimum.

***

That first winter at HM was not what I'd hoped for, but was developing into what I'd feared. Problem after problem kept popping up, and very few of them were attributable to Mum, she was the victim.

Mid-November meant flu jabs for all the residents. This was compulsory and not up for negotiation. I arrived for a visit in the afternoon, having no knowledge that Mum had received the flu vaccination that morning. I located her in the dining room which was at the opposite end of the house from the lounge and joined by a long, wide corridor. She was slumped in a chair by an empty, cavernous fireplace.

The dining room had no heating on at all. My mother was barely conscious and very cold, not only that, she was saturated in urine from her waist down to her slippers and was wearing a makeshift bandage on her head. The sight of her moved me to tears and then a glowing anger started fermenting in the pit of my stomach, not a good sign. Assertiveness was required here, not the full blown rant that my gut was heading towards.

I shouted for a member of staff, who, when she came, was defensive and irritated with me for making a fuss. I was told that the flu jab had been given to everyone that morning, and Joan must have had a slight reaction to it. I pointed out to this slattern that hypothermia was not going to improve Joan's condition and I wanted her cleaned up, warmed up and out of this room.

'Why has she been left in this ice box?' I asked. 'To get this wet and cold she must have been here for hours.'

I could detect the tremble and breathlessness of suppressed anger in my speech.

No, that couldn't be the case, I was assured. They'd used this room for lunch. Lunch was always at 12 noon and it was now 3.30pm.

A wheelchair and an additional member of staff turned up. They proceeded to use an underarm lift, outlawed years ago, as an unacceptable way of lifting anyone unable to bear their own weight. The two of them dragged my mother into the chair, where she slumped over to one side, unresponsive, as they wheeled her to the bedroom. Twenty minutes later they emerged, having changed Mum into her nightdress and put her to bed. I was incensed at what I'd witnessed.

My mother lay in bed, inert and still very cold. Her bedroom was like the inside of a fridge. I touched the radiator, there was no heat from it at all. Later, I was to learn that the heating, throughout the winter, was turned off between 2pm and 5pm in all the rooms except for the lounge.

I went in search of whichever trained nurse was in charge. Unfortunately, it was my least favourite, a big, horsey lady, whose expertise was mental health. I personally felt she would have been better suited as a prison warder.

I confronted her.

'Can you enlighten me as to the purpose of this piece of wadding that's attached to my mother's head?'

As she was now in bed and still wearing it, I presumed it must be serving some purpose. The nurse feigned surprise.

'Hasn't anyone notified you about Joan's fall yesterday?'

She towered over me by some distance and was an intimidating presence. 'No.'

My voice still had that quivering tone of temper, but could have been interpreted as fear of woman, and she might not be able to identify the difference. She explained, as if talking to a three-year-old who'd just asked "why" for the umpteenth time.

Joan had been meandering down the corridor. Another resident with learning difficulties, known for his outbursts and his ability to race around the place to avoid capture, had collided with Joan, or pushed her over. Nobody was sure of the actual facts. She'd cracked her head open on the edge of a door frame.

The doctor had seen her, as yesterday was the day he did his rounds at the nursing home. He didn't feel there was a need to subject her to the stress of going to hospital. The wound had been glued and dressed in-house and they were keeping an eye on it.

I left. I wanted to question the advisability of allowing her to have the flu jab while there was the possibility of concussion but what was the point? The home hadn't seen fit to inform me of any of this. It appeared that I'd forfeited all rights over the care of my own mother the day she entered Huesneath Moor.

***

I painted my lobby on Christmas day that year. A feature wall of squares, using left over tester pots, each square meticulously outlined in gold paint. Maeve Binchy kept me company with her story-telling on talking books bought from the charity shop.

During January, I had a phone call from the vet. A stray cat who answered the description of Missy had been reported living out of dustbins and fighting with indigenous cats. My son's school was situated in the street where the report had originated. The lady who phoned the vet and who was leaving food out for this hobo moggy lived directly opposite the school entrance and only a few hundred yards away from the plumber, who'd gone to such pains to befriend Missy. I went round, delighted at the prospect of a reunion (with Missy, not the plumber).

The lady, whose name was Sarah, was waiting outside for me with the stray cat sitting beside her on a low wall. It was unmistakably Missy. I'd like to report that Mistletoe jumped straight into my waiting arms, but she vehemently resisted the handover and shot off down the road. I was embarrassed at Missy's lack of enthusiasm at the prospect of our reunion. I had to leave it to Sarah to coax her back and between us we eventually completed a rescue. Sarah, upon whom Missy had transferred her affections, couldn't keep her. She had cats of her own that were hell bent on ripping Missy to pieces. Mistletoe had little option but to come home with me.

Once home, it was obvious that the poor little thing was traumatised. Always an introverted and nervous feline, she launched herself out of the carrier, bolted under the kitchen table and refused to come out. I put her bed under there, along with food, water and a litter tray. It was three days before she emerged, having ignored tempting titbits and soft words. Only then could

I examine her properly. There was no doubt she'd had a rough time. Missy was a small cat anyway and now there was no weight to her at all. She was so skinny I could feel her spine, every rib and the scabs and scars of survival on the streets.

Over the next few months she made a complete physical recovery and occasionally ventured through the cat flap into the back garden, but never beyond the boundary wall and never ever near the front door, which she obviously regarded as the gateway to her worst nightmare.

Chapter Eleven

January brought a reduction in staff levels at HM. Although the senior nursing staff remained the same, there was an atmosphere of discontent amongst the care assistants. I suspected it was partly related to the incredibly low pay these girls were getting. The National Minimum Wage law hadn't yet been implemented but employers were being notified as to the implications.

I got the impression that the proprietors of the home were reluctant to replace the girls who'd left, anticipating that they would soon be forced to increase wages at the bottom end of the pay scale. Whatever the reason, members of the care staff were leaving and not being replaced, and the care levels, never brilliant, were suffering as a result. For the most part, I kept my thoughts to myself.

It seemed that Mrs B was becoming less involved. Often I wouldn't see her for days. I wondered if she was finding being at the helm too much to cope with, as she appeared to be delegating more and more to her senior staff.

My mother was deteriorating, though not entirely due to the natural progression of the disease. She only responded to me now as somebody giving her attention, being kind or feeding her with cake. She was unsteady on her feet and spent most of her days in the lounge, huddled in her chair. I never saw anyone attempt to walk her for the benefit of exercising her muscles. It was obvious that soon they'd be too wasted to do the job and anyway her brain would forget how, partly through neglect of this diminishing skill.

I wanted to complain, but there was always the fear that it would rebound on Mum and the staff were obviously under pressure and demoralised. I felt I'd just be shouting into the wind. I watched her with a sense of despair at the inevitable. She sat, isolated in a world of her own, hands moving over invisible objects or stretching out to grasp things unseen to all but her.

Her glasses had been confiscated because she wouldn't keep them on and they had subsequently and mysteriously disappeared. To join her teeth, no doubt. Her hair was no longer permed in the curly style she'd worn all her life, it had been cut short and was worn as a straight, lifeless, institutionalised skull cap. Mum had also lost a great deal of weight which, I was assured when I queried it, was a common characteristic of Alzheimer's.

***

Summer came and I persuaded Margaret that we were both in need of some quality rest and recuperation. Surprisingly she agreed, with minimal reservations, and I booked a week in Tenerife for mid-October. It was intended to be a chill out holiday with minimal exertion. The weather was on our side with wall to wall sunshine for the entire week.

71

We took the obligatory coach trip to Mount Teide and a few bus rides to various other parts of the island, including the famous Loro Parque with its amazing penguinarium. We were staying at Puerto de la Cruz which was a wonderful town to walk through in the evening. Unlike some of the resorts in the south of the island, Puerto de la Cruz had a local feel, with families out and about, eating al fresco or meandering through the plazas, enjoying the balmy evenings and the street entertainment.

One day, we decided to take the local bus to Santa Cruz, just to say we'd seen Tenerife's capital city. I'd been unwell during the night due to a slight upset stomach. The suspected culprit was the lunch I'd eaten the day before during a visit to a resort in the south of the island, but I thought I was fit enough for this excursion.

Once on the bus, I felt woozy and knew I was about to pass out. I faint fairly easily. I can sometimes prevent it if I can get my head down between my knees, but in the bus there wasn't enough room to do that. I passed out, head slumped forward onto the back of the seat in front.

Margaret, not a natural nurse, thought I was asleep and so left me alone until we were nearing our destination. She roused me with difficulty. Because I'd been out of it for sometime, my blood pressure had plummeted through my boots and I struggled to function. I staggered off the bus into the bus station and collapsed on the nearest bench. The world was spinning around me and I was unable to move from my horizontal position.

I knew what had happened and explained the situation to Margaret. I was just going to have to wait it out. I certainly wouldn't be doing any sightseeing. I wasn't even well enough to get back on a bus and wouldn't be for some hours. There was undoubtedly a hint of recrimination, that Margaret hadn't recognised what had happened and made an attempt to bring me round sooner.

Margaret, always the pragmatist, decided to sightsee on her own.

'Do you mind? Will you be all right here on your own?' she asked.

Yes, I did mind and no, I wouldn't be all right, would have been the correct response, but there wasn't a great deal she could do. I was drifting in and out of sleep, so not scintillating company.

She left me, sprawled out on the bench in the bus station, like some bag lady, while she disappeared for what seemed like hours. I was desperate to use the toilet and needed fluids but couldn't remain upright long enough to accomplish either.

Margaret assured me that she really enjoyed the experience. There was a small gauge train that took her around the port and a park. A large cruise liner had just berthed, spilling out a crowd of English speaking tourists, so she just went along with the crowd and their tour guide. Margaret has always possessed the enviable ability to be able to converse with just about anyone.

When she returned, Margaret bought me a cup of tea from a vendor within the bus station, who I'd viewed, gagging with thirst, from my bench, but had been too wobbly to get to. By mid-afternoon I'd recovered enough to risk walking the few steps to the bus. Once back at the hotel, I forfeited dinner for bed and slept for twelve straight hours.

It was a story retold at every opportunity and embellished with each telling. How my best friend, who couldn't tell the difference between sleep and unconsciousness, had left me alone in a bus station for hours although I was ill and possibly dying, while she went off on a sightseeing tour.

***

November arrived and so did the dreaded flu vaccination programme. Whether it was an adverse reaction to the flu jab, I couldn't say, but Joan became ill within hours of receiving the vaccination. She couldn't be roused and within twenty-four hours she was full of congestion, which rattled ominously in her chest. The nurse on duty was sufficiently concerned to ring me at home to inform me that my mother was seriously ill. The doctor had diagnosed pneumonia.

I sat by her bed, listening to her laboured breathing, her hand limp and unresponsive within my grasp. I thought that this was the end and part of me was relieved. My mother's quality of life was so impoverished and the general care levels at HM were inadequate at best. Strangely, now that she was near to death, the staff couldn't do enough for her. What a contradiction, I thought. Presented with the challenge of someone with severe dementia, now at death's door, they're falling over each other to keep her alive.

I even attributed their new found zeal to the fact that at the start of the winter months beds began to empty as colds, flu and pneumonia took their toll. By January, the local Health Authority had often run out of money to fund replacement people for the empty beds. They wouldn't receive their new financial allocation until April. In a bad year, care staff had to be laid off.

On the way home, I drove into the most beautiful sunset, a few hilltop houses and trees silhouetted black against a red sky. I was consumed with the turmoil of conflicting thoughts and images of my mother who would be unable to appreciate this scene. Not now, not ever again in this life, whether she lived or died. What did I want for her, to live or rest in death? I wanted the latter, but knew I'd never do anything to bring it about. Like the staff at the home, I would fight for her life, just as they were doing. I pulled into the lay-by and wept until there were no more tears and no more thought, just the chill of the night and the serenity of the quiet darkness and a heart that had become reconciled.

Against all the odds, my mother survived the pneumonia followed by septicaemia, but during the prolonged period in bed, she forgot how to walk and would never again stand upright or bear her own weight.

Around the same time Mrs B told me that she was going to retire and was handing the reins over to a manager in the New Year.

***

Christmas 1999 came and went. Missy and I spent most of it curled up on the settee with a good book and comfort food (chocolates and toffee-flavoured popcorn) augmented by extra shifts at work.

New Year's Eve at Bideford attracted people from far and wide. It was reputed as being the place to be after Edinburgh and Trafalgar Square. The ancient Bideford Long Bridge which spanned the River Torridge with its twenty four pointed arches was within shouting distance of my cottage.

The bridge featured large in the celebration. Though I'd never been part of it, I was given to understand that, on the first stroke of midnight, the celebrants attempted to race from the west side to the east side of the bridge and back again, before Big Ben completed its twelve bongs. This was immediately followed by the brave, or foolhardy, climbing the parapet of the bridge and jumping into the river (tides permitting) though I suspect Health and Safety regulations have put a stop to that these days.

I watched the firework display from my garden, impressive starbursts engulfing the sky above my head. This was the big one, the beginning of the first year of the new century. Many hoped it would bring peace and prosperity, whilst doom mongers prophesied that this new millennium would be heralded by every computerised system failing and planes falling out of the sky. Between the Christmas and New Year I became fifty. An utterly depressing week.

***

My first visit to Huesneath Moor in January 2000 was to cement the trend for that year. I was told by the staff that they now had a manager, Brian. His background was in mental health rather than geriatric or general nursing, so I was prepared to be less than impressed. It was the end of February before I actually met the man, and by then I was beginning to feel that even my low expectations about care levels were not being met.

Mum had been confined to her room since she'd lost the use of her legs. The reason for this varied depending on who I spoke to, but eventually they settled on the official explanation. Joan had become very vocal and it distressed the other residents. My mother, it seemed, now screamed and shouted from morning until night, only stopping to eat. Admittedly, I could hear her the minute I entered the building and it was top volume.

'Hasn't Brian, our resident psychiatric expert, got any theories as to why my mother screams so much?' I said, with more than a hint of sarcasm.

My question was met with a little raising of the eyes and a little raising of the hands, in unison. Apparently, Brian wasn't overly hands-on, busy hatching plans in his office, by all accounts.

Whatever the theories, the facts were that Mum was spending the entire winter in her bedroom, which, social deprivation apart, was akin to living in an igloo. The room in which a resident spends his or her day should be heated to provide a constant level of warmth of twenty degrees centigrade. That was not the case in Joan's room. The heating went off altogether between 2pm and 5pm. The radiators, which had protective covers that masked the heat, were struggling to warm the room to anywhere near a comfortable temperature. I took in a room thermometer on several occasions and parked it, out of sight, for the time I was there. Even in my coat, I always felt chilled

74

by the time I went home and the thermometer reading never came close to the twenty degree mark.

After numerous complaints, which were totally ignored, I reported the home to Registration, the inspectorate which upheld the rules and regulations appertaining to nursing and residential homes. They did an unannounced spot check, on a mild, sunny day and found the room to be adequately heated.

My mother's bedroom had two outside walls, which provided a lot of windows. It made the room cold on dull winter days but warm when the sun was shining through the glass. A lottery I'd failed to win. Registration, of course, couldn't really afford to find too many faults with any one home, especially when there were only two EMI units in a large chunk of Devon. Where on earth would they put all this frail humanity if they were forced to close one of them?

I resorted to Plan B, which entailed asking if an additional form of heating could be put in Mum's room.

'No,' was the reply from their illustrious manager, 'because a trailing lead poses a hazard. The resident using the room might trip.'

I pointed out the blindingly obvious, that she was incapable of standing up, never mind tripping over anything. I was sure the furniture could be arranged in such a way that the lead would pose a minimal risk. This conversation with Brian wasn't face to face, but through the intermediary services of a care assistant.

I had to sign a disclaimer, and the additional heater was provided, though its benefits to my mother did depend on a member of staff switching it on, which didn't always happen.

***

Within the constraints of my work timetable, I was now varying the times of my visits, so that staff couldn't so easily anticipate my arrival. Such was the level of disquiet I felt at the care being given to Joan. She was losing so much weight that I found it difficult to believe that it was entirely due to Alzheimer's. It was much more symptomatic of malnutrition.

My mother was no longer going to the dining room for meals, but was being fed in her room by a care assistant. She relied on staff to give her any drinks as she wasn't able to hold a cup or feed herself.

On one of these unscheduled visits, I found Mum in her room and on the floor. She had an ordinary armchair and would slide downwards. Being unable to pull herself upright, she would continue to slide until the carpet blocked her progress. Straps or harnesses to secure people like Joan, into chairs, had been prohibited in recent years, deemed to be undue restraint. I viewed her plight, of being free to slide onto the floor, as a contravention of health and safety, but the rule book didn't agree. I approached senior staff with a solution.

'The way around this problem,' I said, 'is for me to provide a reclining chair, so that being in a reclined position to begin with, Mum will be much less likely to keep sliding onto the floor.'

'No,' was the answer, 'because if Joan isn't able to get out of the chair and in a reclined position she wouldn't be able to, that is termed as undue restraint.'

I lost it.

'This is total madness.' I said. 'I want her to have a reclining chair so at least she is comfortable in that position, instead of reclining on a hard floor because she isn't checked on often enough. Give me a disclaimer, or whatever I have to sign, to make this happen *today*.'

My loss of composure was regrettable but I was presented with something to sign, which I did, with steam emanating from my ears.

It didn't happen that day, of course, because I had to go and buy one and then arrange for it to be delivered to the home. But within a week Mum was settled into her pink recliner. I'd like to say that this was the last battle I had to fight on her behalf, but it was only the start.

***

Joan was constantly developing urinary tract infections. These would send her downhill very fast, becoming unresponsive and generally unwell with a raised temperature. I suggested that she wasn't being given anywhere near enough to drink. Tucked away in her room all day, she was easily overlooked, in spite of the shouting.

My mother was in fine fettle, however, one day during the summer, when she had a visit from her sister, Barbara. She'd previously visited Joan a few weeks before her eviction from Mount Kingsley, eighteen months ago. Her sister had now changed out of all recognition and nothing I could have said would have adequately prepared Barbara. But Mum was having a good day, with no screaming and she even managed a smile in response to her sister's cajoling.

Chapter Twelve

Joan no longer had control over her bladder and leaked urine constantly and her bowel movements were in response to suppositories. She'd had a lifelong combative relationship with her bowel. She was the "Senna Queen", the normal action of her intestines shot to pieces through the overuse of laxatives. But incontinence of urine was becoming a contentious problem.

I made an unexpected morning visit to find that somebody had put a wheelchair cushion on the seat of my mother's chair, as a makeshift waterproof barrier. She'd slipped downwards on the shiny surface of the cushion so that her body was on the extended part of the chair and her legs, below the knees, were dangling over the end of the recliner, her head resting on the wet wheelchair cushion. I flipped.

I was so angry that the red mist had developed a maroon hue. I trounced into the lounge and demanded to see Brian. I wanted him to witness the level of care my mother was getting. Predictably, he wasn't on duty. A senior member of staff, Louise, who'd reassured me the day I brought Mum to HM, walked me back to my mother's room where two care staff scurried to put things right, fixing the damage. Frustration was threatening to dissolve into tears and I really didn't want to lose control.

Louise sat with me in Mum's room, after harmony had been restored and the care staff had disappeared. She vented her frustration at the patchy care that was on offer. She said that Brian was beginning to make changes, but his efforts were being met with resistance from some staff, the ones who'd enjoyed an easy ride for too long. Wages had been increased at the lower end of the scale and it was now felt that staff had to become more professional in their approach. Brian was going to bring Joan back into the lounge for a couple of hours, during the mornings. He felt that her noise levels were probably exacerbated by being isolated in her room.

'You don't have to be Einstein to work that one out,' I said.

Louise agreed it was an obvious conclusion, but to the staff, it would mean extra work, and they didn't want to acknowledge the benefits Joan would receive.

Louise asked me about the things that Joan had particularly enjoyed before her illness. I thought about it for a while. It was difficult to cast my mind back to before dementia. My mother had always been up for a laugh, never averse to acting the fool. She was the antithesis of my father, who was an introverted man, uncomfortable in social situations with unfamiliar people. Mum liked music, not classical, but the popular tunes of her day and into the 1960s and 1970s.

'She loved babies,' I added. I made the statement as if I'd uncovered the Holy Grail.

It was true, Mum had enjoyed being with children, always at ease and able to get on their wavelength, but she adored babies. I found a tiny bundle of baby daunting and never felt comfortable holding one, I didn't know what it expected of me and always felt that I'd failed to deliver. It was invariably a self-fulfilling prophecy, because the baby would feel the tension and start to bawl. Mum was a natural with babies and yearned to hold them, change them, feed them, coo and converse with them.

Louise made the suggestion that I brought in a baby doll for Joan. There were some brilliant ones around, life-size and so realistic. I'd momentarily panicked on more than one occasion, seeing young children swinging these dolls by one arm or careering across the park at breakneck speed with a pushchair containing a baby doll. Louise felt a doll might have a calming effect on Joan, something she could relate to on some level. It was certainly worth a try.

All this one to one attention had the desired effect of bringing me down off the ceiling. Louise was an expert at the oil pouring process and she did make me feel that I had an ally.

The wheelchair cushion incident would not be repeated, Louise assured me, but good care practices weren't going to happen overnight. Brian intended to set up in-house training for staff, to bring their skills up to present day standards, but it would all take time.

***

I went home reassured, but that false sense of security wasn't to last for long. I still attended monthly meetings for carers of people with Alzheimer's disease and was sad when I was told, at the meeting, that the group was disbanding as there wasn't sufficient support to warrant the cost of hiring the room. It was at this final get together that I heard the rumour, from a care manager of a local residential home. Mum's nursing home was up for sale.

I decided to shelve the rumour for the time being, after all that's all it was, a rumour. One person who said she thought Huesneath Moor was to be sold.

Joan was moved into the lounge during the mornings and remained there until lunchtime or until her noise levels became unacceptable to the majority. The baby doll had some success. At times she clung onto it when it was placed in her arms, at other times the unnervingly lifelike doll was left neglected and ignored. Whether it gave Joan some level of comfort or not, was inconclusive.

The upside was, it attracted a good deal of attention from staff, visitors and other residents, who all desired to get their hands on it, to rearrange its clothes, disrobe it, dress it in alternative attire, cradle it and talk to my mother about it. So from that obscure angle it was very successful indeed.

By the end of the summer, I hadn't seen any other signs of improved care levels. The first thing I had to do on virtually every visit was to ask staff to change Mum because she'd be soaked in urine, often necessitating a complete change of clothing.

Conversely, I wasn't happy about the amount of fluids she was being given. If Joan wasn't drinking enough, the bladder would become irritated leading to a constant leaking of urine which never fully emptied the bladder, but left a pool of stagnant urine behind that became a breeding ground for bacterial infection. Joan's plight was quite likely to be primarily due to damage caused by the dementia, but it was also symptomatic of insufficient fluid intake, aggravated by lack of staff training. This was a nursing home and this was basic nursing care, but if care staff hadn't been taught, it wasn't going to happen.

***

An afternoon visit in late September was met with the usual soggy mother and the habitual request, by me, for her to be changed. Most of the staff were on a tea break, but one care assistant offered to change Mum, if I could assist with the hoist, to move her from the chair to the bed. I was happy to do that, though I was aware that I shouldn't have been asked, nor should I have been involved in the use of the hoist. I was trained, but as a visitor, not a member of staff, I wasn't covered by insurance should an accident occur. It was obvious that this care assistant had no procedural knowledge and therefore I doubted that she'd undergone any proper training in the use of this bit of kit.

Once my mother was on the bed, the care assistant proceeded to remove wet clothes and pad. I noticed, to my horror, that she had extensive urine burns to her groin and buttocks. How I didn't explode I don't know. I think I managed to hold it together, because I wanted to see how the care assistant would react. She didn't. She simply replaced the wet pad with a dry one. No washing and barrier creaming of the inflamed skin was done at all. I was stunned into silence.

This was serious neglect and not something that had happened overnight. It was the result of bad practice over a prolonged period. Losing my rag wasn't an option, this complaint had to be dealt with properly. I put my concerns in writing, initially to Louise.

The staff appeared to be divided into two teams. That was an observation on my part, not necessarily a fact, but then facts were thin on the ground at the nursing home. There appeared to be two trained nurses taking the lead, during the day. Louise, a state registered nurse and Katrina, who was a psychiatric nurse and not a lady I'd ever warmed to. There was also Rachel, who seemed very caring, but was not there as often. I presumed she was a bank nurse who filled in for off-duty staff, those on holiday and any of the workforce on sick leave.

After I'd completed my night shifts, I took in the letter on my next visit. Louise was on holiday for another week and I felt that this situation couldn't go on unchecked. Rachel was in charge, so I voiced my concerns to her and gave her the letter. She promised to ensure that Louise received the letter and asked me if I had any preference as to what cream was to be used on Joan's sore flesh. I couldn't quite believe I'd been asked that question by a trained nurse. I drew her attention to the full tub of barrier cream in Mum's room and said, that as far as I was concerned it was as good as anything else, certainly better than nothing and available for use now.

'But if you know of a cream that's more effective, please let me know and I'll provide it,' I added.

I was trying to keep my voice even and not convey the anger that was simmering within. A care assistant, who was hovering on the periphery of this conversation, informed me that the manager and staff were already aware of the problem and Joan's care notes reflected that fact. It'd been a problem since March. Joan was also, she stated, on bed rest in the afternoons, without a pad, to aid the healing process.

That little speech was almost my undoing. My mother hadn't been in bed on my last visit, which had been in the afternoon. She'd suffered this neglect for six months or more and action was only being taken now, because I'd inadvertently seen the damage and they were pre-empting my complaint to Brian, or more likely afraid that I'd make a report to Registration.

A week later, I received a phone call from Louise, who apologised for the inexcusable discomfort and pain that Joan had suffered for so long and confirmed my assessment that it was urine burn. She confessed to finding it difficult to get all care staff and a particular member of the nursing staff, to follow preventative procedures. She asked me if I would be prepared to make a formal complaint to the manager, Brian. Louise felt my complaint would be supporting her and she'd welcome a bit of support right now.

On my next two visits, I found that Mum was indeed on bed rest in the afternoon, but on both occasions she was lying in a wet bed. During this period, I had a long talk to Louise, who was feeling very frustrated because care plans weren't being followed by all the staff and therefore it was difficult to get on top of Joan's problem. She told me that a certain member of the nursing staff habitually re-used pads that were soiled. Louise was so disillusioned with care standards that she would welcome my intervention at any level, even reporting it to Registration.

***

On my next visit, I asked to see Brian and explained all my concerns to him. I told him, that on a general level, I felt the basic nursing care was very poor. Every time I visited, the first thing I had to do for my mother was clean the caked yellow matter off her eyes and clean the build up of wax from her outer ears and ask the staff to change her urine soaked pad and clothes. I was extremely concerned about my recent discovery of urine burn to her buttocks and groin and to me it pointed to several possibilities:
1. Joan was being left in urine soaked pads and clothes for too long.
2. She wasn't being washed and creamed when she was changed.
3. She wasn't given sufficient fluids.
4. Joan was having urine soiled pads put back on.

I made it clear that I thought all these possibilities applied in my mother's case and also added that I regarded bed rest in the afternoon as being less than useless, as she was being left to lie in a wet bed.

Brian admitted that care levels were a problem and there were some staff that he wished could be dispensed with. As a registered mental nurse in a nursing home for the EMI, his first priority had been to rectify some of the glaring problems in the area of mental health. He felt perhaps, as his new policies inevitably meant staff had to give more time to that side of care, nursing levels had probably dropped as a result. It was a predicament he now had to get on top of. He appeared to accept what I said and told me he would set up a fluid chart for Joan, to ensure sufficient intake.

When I returned four days later there was no evidence of a fluid chart. Louise, the nurse on duty that afternoon, knew nothing about it, or about my conversation with the manager. She said she would speak to Brian and ensure a fluid chart was set up. She phoned me later to say that she'd done both. The manager had apologised for not talking to her before. He'd been too busy.

On my next visit, I noted that the bottles of cordial were still not being used at a reasonable rate and there was still no fluid chart to be found. Charts of this kind were usually kept in the room, though not on display, so that the amount of fluid can be recorded at the time it's given and signed by the person giving it. I queried the absence of a chart with a care assistant, who told me that all such charts were kept in the office, and she did show me my mother's chart. I didn't feel reassured, as a care worker myself, I know how easy it is to get sidetracked. By the time you got to the office, it would, at best, be a guesstimate, at worst, a complete work of fiction, if it was done at all.

By the time I left HM that day, I'd made two decisions. To look for another nursing home for Mum and to keep a record of any further incidents rather than rely on my memory, just in case. In case of what, I wasn't sure at this point.

***

I'd booked a holiday in Italy, a small village in the Dolomite Mountains. I was in dire need of a break and the trip was a last minute deal and was by coach all the way. Never again. Coach travel is fine, but even when I'd travelled to Scotland there had been an overnight stopover in Leeds. This was a recipe for deep vein thrombosis.

My fellow travellers could be divided into three groups. The stalwart walkers equipped with Nordic poles and the appropriate footwear. A party of friends who liked the idea of being stuck in a hotel in the mountains with nothing to do all day except drink and look out at the view. And an elderly lady who was having difficulty getting on and off the coach for the toilet stops. What she thought she was going to do halfway up the Dolomites, I couldn't say and I think she was beginning to wish she'd done a little more research. I was the floating voter, unsure where to pledge my allegiance. I'd come with a cagoule, trainers and a sketch pad.

The mountain scenery was worth the trip, whatever the motive. Stunning didn't come close. I tagged onto the seasoned walkers, who had maps of the trails, but soon realised that I didn't have the stamina or the equipment to be taken as a serious walker. They were all incredibly kind, but I was obviously holding them back.

I decided to go for a walk on my own using a map in one of the brochures from the hotel's reception desk. What could go wrong? It was a warm day with the hint of autumn in the air and on the leaves of the deciduous trees. I ignored the fact that I'm notorious for having no sense of direction.

The trail markers were attached to trees and for the first two hours I followed the trail through the mountain forest, stopping to take photographs. In a clearing where trees had been felled and the logs were stacked ready for transportation off the mountain, I sat down on a log pile and ate my packed lunch.

After devouring my crisps, chocolate bar and a somewhat pappy apple, I started on the route back to my hotel, or so I thought. Scenery always looks totally different from the opposite direction, so I wasn't alerted by the fact that nothing seemed familiar. Half an hour of brisk walking and I was beginning to wonder where the trail markers had gone. I'd no idea where I was. What now? Well, I reasoned, it was a trail so it must lead somewhere. I don't know what I was expecting. These were the Dolomites, I was hardly going to come to a clearing and find McDonalds and a Travelodge.

The trail came to an abrupt halt at a clearing where the forest gave way to a grassy slope, so steep that a narrow path had been dug into the side of the hill. The path would aid a mountain goat to get to the other side, but a middle-aged lady in a cagoule and trainers? I glanced at the sky. The sun was low and dusk was approaching. Halfway along the narrow track, walking foot in front of foot, clutching onto the grassy slope rising above me, the thought struck me that I hadn't told anyone where I was going. Nobody would know where to even begin to search and if I lost my footing now I was going to die.

I reached the other side of the clearing where the trail resumed and slumped to the ground until I'd stopped shaking. The forest had become gloomy, but if I stuck to the trail, I'd be okay. What was the worst that could happen? I might have to spend the night in the forest. I quickened my step, still hoping to arrive at civilisation before nightfall. My screams bounced off the trees as a deer broke through the undergrowth and leapt across the path in front of me. It was at that point I decided that a night in the forest was not the benign option I'd envisaged.

It was dark by the time the trail led me to a few houses and a road. I recognised it as being at the top of Fondo, the village where I was staying. I could see the lights of the hotel below me. I had to walk another half a mile down to the hotel, but I'd survived. I was greeted with cheers as I went through the door into the bar. The owner gave me a scolding for not informing him where I'd intended going that day. I accepted the dressing down, too relieved to even think of excuses.

I stuck to organised coach trips for the rest of the holiday. I could get lost just as easily in Bolzano or Verona.

The holiday had re-energised me, so it was a feistier fighter for human rights who arrived at HM to see my mother on the 26th October. It was an afternoon visit just before my first night back at work. A cup of tea had been placed in Mum's room, but nobody had helped her to drink it, and as usual she hadn't been given any cake. Everyone else received a slice of cake with their afternoon cup of tea, except my mother, because it took five minutes to feed it to her. There were four members of staff standing around chatting together, I asked for cake and a warm cup of tea. While I was feeding Mum and giving her a blow by blow account of my Italian holiday I noticed that her fingernails were like talons and contained suspicious debris. I usually cut them because it's easier to do the job myself than have to make an additional complaint, but having been away, it had been well over a month since they'd been done and I hadn't brought my clippers with me.

Her trousers and the plastic backed incontinence pad that kept the chair dry were both damp, so I asked that Mum be changed. That request was met with a protest from three of the four members of staff who were gathered together.

'She was only changed ten minutes before you arrived,' said one of the carers.

'That might be the case and her pad might not be wet, but her trousers and the pad she's sitting on certainly are, and my mother needs changing,' I replied.

Two care assistants came in to do the job they were paid for, one of whom was still complaining.

'It's probably sweat,' she said.

'It smells like urine to me,' I replied.

The staff discovered that the protective chair pad no longer had a waterproof backing and the chair beneath it was wet, therefore urine had leaked upwards through the pad that was no longer fit for purpose.

At that point I was beginning to lose all pretence at remaining calm under fire. I wanted to shout and gesticulate menacingly so I walked out of the room until I'd forced the destructive emotion back into its box.

Having regained some semblance of calm, I went back into my mother's room. She'd been moved into her other armchair and there was no evidence of a wheelchair or hoist in the room. It didn't take much imagination to visualise how they'd transferred her from one chair to the other.

The next day, I had a phone call from Mrs B, the owner of the home. She said she'd been given to understand that I'd been upset by the confrontational attitude of a member of her staff. Mrs B felt this was intolerable and would I be prepared to make a written complaint. I told her that I'd already drafted a letter to the manager and I would be coming in with my brother on the 1st November to give Brian the letter and hopefully speak to him. We went on to talk about our mutual concerns about care levels. It was Mrs B's opinion that one or two individuals are responsible for the problems.

I hadn't been strictly honest with Mrs B. The draft letter was still in my head and not on paper. I have a rule for complaints. I always allow three days before putting pen to paper, a cooling-off period where I mull it over. On the third day, if I'm still seething or feel a letter should be sent because it's the right thing to do, then I transfer the draft letter in my brain onto paper. After three days I was still seething and it definitely was the right thing to do.

I have a system for letters of complaint. I always begin with commendation where I can. The softening-up process.

I wrote that I had noticed an improvement in some areas of Joan's care that I'd previously voiced concerns about. Her eyes and ears were much cleaner and Louise informed me that the urine burns to her bottom and groin have now cleared, for which I was grateful.

Then I socked it to them!

However, I wrote, *I'm still concerned about aspects of basic care that I feel are not being met adequately.*

I allowed this initial statement to lead into a detailed account of my version of events. I then moved to the empathy strategy, followed by the veiled implication that I might take this further.

I do appreciate the problems you're faced with and I'm not unsympathetic, but this is my mother and these are not, I feel, unrealistic or unreasonable concerns, because there are basic nursing standards for the elderly and they are not being met. Mum doesn't require much more than the basics, given adequate food and fluids, kept clean, warm and dry and treated with TLC, but some of these basic requirements are time consuming and that, I suspect, is where the problem lies.

Chapter Thirteen

Bob came with me on my next visit to HM. Katrina, the Registered Mental Nurse in charge who was also on duty on the 26th October, came into Mum's room to see us. She had her non-confrontational face on, as well she might. I reckoned that she was high on the list of Mrs B's suspects. I gave her the letter for the manager and stressed my hope that we would be able to see him that day.

'Unfortunately Brian is out and not due back until 5pm. Is this about the chair incident?' she asked.

'Yes, amongst other things,' I replied.

She asked if everything was in order today. My answer was noncommittal as I'd only just arrived and hadn't had time to assess the situation. I did notice that one and a half bottles of cordial had been used in a period of five days, which was better than usual, but Mum's eyes were caked with yellow discharge, her ears needed cleaning and her fingernails still hadn't been cut.

Five days later, Brian hadn't been in touch with me with reference to the letter. On my next visit on 5th November, I took my nail clippers with me and cut Mum's nails.

Vicky again apologised for the events of the 26th October, which I appreciated. She admitted that she'd asked for a transfer to the other care team, because she was fed up with the care levels administered by Katrina's team. She said that care staff were quite prepared to sit around doing crosswords and reading magazines when there was work that needed to be done and she'd made a formal complaint to management.

The wheelchair cushion had reappeared on the recliner, no doubt to prevent the chair from getting wet and a cheaper option than investing in new seat pads, but inevitably it will make it easier for Mum to slide down onto the floor. Two packets of jellies and twelve chocolate bars had been eaten, supposedly by my mother, in five days. If they gave her a drink every time she (or they) consumed her sweets, she would be getting adequate fluids.

***

The next day, I decided to kickstart my plan to move Mum out of HM. I rang Age Concern at the office local to the nursing home. I spoke to a member of the team there. He said that my concerns were not the only ones they'd received, in connection with this particular nursing home. He asked me if I knew that the home was up for sale. He said he'd seen it advertised as a potential conference centre and felt that care levels were unlikely to improve and I'd do well to look elsewhere for a nursing home for my mother. He promised to mention my concerns to her GP when he next saw him on the

10th November.

I rang Brian to see if he'd received my letter. He said he'd only just come back from leave that day. He would write to me outlining point by point what he intended to do.

9th November, 2000

Dear Jill,

Thank you for your letter of the 30th October, and I am sorry for the delay in getting back to you.

I am also sorry that you have concerns about your mother's care here at Huesneath Moor. You raise a number of issues in your letter and I will deal with them separately if you don't mind.

In saying that, the matter of the cordial and the finger nails are connected. We are having great difficulty getting it through to staff that if they see something needs doing to go ahead and do it and not assume someone else will. To counteract this mindset I am in the process of creating a new key worker system that will mean that care assistants will be accountable for the care of individual residents, so things such as nails will be their responsibility. The resident's family will be informed of who the care worker is so that they know who to discuss day to day matters of care with. Getting the right care assistant with the right resident is not an easy one as I am sure you can imagine, but I hope to have it in place before the end of November. This will improve basic care as it will mean that staff will no longer be able to blame someone else.

Moving and handling is an issue that we are also addressing with a training session on 22nd November, after this staff will have no excuse for any bad practice.

Your mother's incontinence and its effect on both her physical and mental state is one of our major concerns at the moment. I have spoken to Dr A (Joan's GP) about this as well. Your mother appears to have reached the stage of total incontinence, in that there is a constant trickle of urine. Recently your mother was changed six times in three hours. Untrained staff have difficulty accepting this can happen, although that is no excuse for any confrontational attitude. I am concerned about how this is affecting your mother, especially as her noise levels have increased. Fluids are being pushed even though there may have been very little evidence as such. Fluid charts were kept for a short while and these showed that your mother was averaging two litres a day, well above the minimum requirement. In my discussion with Dr A we talked about catheterisation, this will help her, both physically and mentally. Louise also feels this may be our best option of care but we would like your views on this before we go ahead with it.

The confrontational attitude of some of the staff has been addressed by both me and the Owners and staff have been made aware that it will not be tolerated. I can only apologise for their behaviour.

I know you are aware of some of the difficulties I face here and thank you and your brother for your support and patience.

During my next visit, I asked Louise for her views on catheterisation. She was in favour of going ahead with it. She felt it would help to prevent the re-occurrence of urine burn and would encourage staff to increase Joan's fluid levels. All sound reasoning, which was swaying my viewpoint, until she dropped the bombshell.

My only ally in the home, Louise, was about to hand in her notice the next day, so she wouldn't be around to oversee things. Catheterisation was a sterile and invasive procedure and so far I'd seen little evidence of competence in any area of nursing care at Huesneath Moor. I also heard that Katrina, whose team appeared to be responsible for most of the problems, was having an affair with the manager, Brian. I felt there was now an urgent need to explore other options as I'd totally lost faith in this nursing home as a care provider.

When I returned home I rang a nursing home in Braunton and had a long chat with the matron there. She was appalled that Joan had been left without glasses and teeth (which happened within the first six months). She said that it constituted abuse. The matron was sympathetic, but regretted that Joan's shouting would be an issue.

'It's gone on for so long without being dealt with, it's probably become a habit that will be difficult to correct. I have to think of the impact on my other residents,' she said.

I contacted another large home, reputed to have good levels of nursing care. It wouldn't have been appropriate when I had to move Mum from Mount Kingsley, but she no longer posed a threat to other residents and good nursing care was the priority. I was told by their receptionist that there was a waiting list, but that the matron would ring me back. She didn't.

I also phoned Registration to ascertain if there was any current legislation that would ensure the nursing home retained its usage when it was sold. Apparently, the owners were under no obligation to sell it as a nursing home. Prospective buyers would be able to apply for change of use, to whatever they required.

On my next visit to HM with Bob, I took in the letter of acceptance for the catheterisation procedure to go ahead. It'd already been done. I left the letter for Brian anyway.

***

On the way home in the car, Bob was unusually quiet and tight lipped. He hated the visits to HM and was also struggling with his own problems. Marie had developed an extreme love affair with alcohol which was now a major problem for which there appeared to be no easy answer.

We were now faced with the prospect of finding new accommodation for Mum, a situation we could no longer ignore and needed to resolve sooner rather than later. Staff were already starting to leave the sinking ship. I decided to share my embryonic plan with Bob.

'I could do it, you know,' I said, 'it's been on my mind for a while.'

There was a pause while the statement was digested.

'I don't think that's a good idea, it nearly broke you last time.'

The words were adamant, the tone less so. I risked a further foray into uncharted territory.

'This is different. The level of care needed now is the type of work I'm familiar with. I've been doing it for years. I'd do a far better job than the nursing home. I've enquired about alternative homes, but the ones I think are any good either won't take her or there's a waiting list. If the home gets sold, we won't have a choice, Mum will just be dumped anywhere that'll have her.'

Bob didn't tell me I was talking rubbish, he didn't say anything for a long time.

'You know I'd support you anyway I could, but I can't be hands-on,' he said finally.

'I wouldn't expect you to be,' I replied. 'But it won't be a cheap option. We'll need to find a suitable place to live, a bungalow obviously and kit it out. I'd have to buy in care to give me some time off, plus the cost of respite care and day to day living expenses. It will all add up. If I did some initial costing, could you take over the financial side of it? I don't think I could cope with that.'

Another prolonged silence.

'We should've hung on to Mum's bungalow. You won't make that mistake with your cottage will you?'

I'd foreseen these two issues coming up.

'The layout in Mum's place would have been useless for wheelchair access and it had a shower room, which won't be any good to her now. As for my place, I know you think I'd be making a bad judgement call, but yes, I would sell it. I've put a lot of work into that little cottage, it's an old place and needs a lot of ongoing TLC. I couldn't bear to leave it in the hands of tenants who wouldn't look after it. I'd rather sell it and walk away.'

By the time we reached home, we were both in a more positive frame of mind than we'd been for months. We had the skeleton of a plan. It felt as if we were taking back control. It was liberating.

***

What we were proposing to do by taking Mum out of a nursing home and into my care was not an unprecedented action but was certainly an unusual one. As a care worker, I'd never personally encountered this situation or even heard about it second hand. We were unsure of where to start.

Common sense told us that just to roll up at HM and tell them that I was taking Joan into my care wouldn't, or shouldn't, be allowed. Social Services seemed to think otherwise.

I rang them with my proposal and was put through by a bemused employee to Ms M. She saw no reason to be concerned and seemed to think that as next of kin I could do what I liked. I felt the need to play devil's advocate. I argued that they ought to be concerned as my mother was a vulnerable adult. I could be planning to deviously shorten her life for the inheritance. I also queried Social Services' role in this proposal. Shouldn't they at least assess her needs to ascertain if I could meet them? Obviously out of her depth, but not willing to concede that I had a valid point, she told me that her boss, Mr Jones, would ring me the next day.

I contacted The Alzheimer's Society for advice. Their legal beagle told me in no uncertain terms that Social Services had a duty of care and should prevent me from taking my mother out of the nursing home until they'd assessed her needs. Social Services needed to be confident that I could provide a level of care that equalled, preferably bettered, that of her present care provider. In effect, they should be working for Joan.

Chapter Fourteen

I visited HM on the morning of the 20th November and although she wasn't shouting and it was mid-morning Mum was in her room, rather than the lounge. Vicky, her proposed care worker under Brian's new scheme, told me that she'd handed in her notice. This meant both Louise and Vicky, the only two members of staff I had any faith in, were both leaving. Morale at the home was at rock bottom.

The next day, Mr Jones from Social Services rang. He was unhelpful to a degree that beggared belief. He took the same line as Ms M and said that as Joan's next of kin, there was no problem. I was free to take her out of Huesneath Moor. His only suggestion was that I get in touch with my mother's GP. I rang off very disgruntled. If what he'd told me was true, then the system was wrong, on so many levels.

I made an appointment to speak to Dr A, Mum's GP. It was the first time I'd met him and was relieved to find that he was a fatherly figure, approachable and easy to talk to. However, he wasn't in favour of me taking my mother out of the nursing home. He certainly had the measure of the place, and nothing he told me inspired confidence that care levels would improve there. He'd been reluctant to catheterise Joan, but all his requests for more frequent changes of pad and clothes were ignored, and in the end he felt he was left with little option. A different story from Brian's interpretation of events.

Dr A's negative reaction to my proposal was to do with the impact it would have on my life. He felt that my mother was so much within a world of her own now, she wasn't as adversely affected by the indifferent care she received as I imagined. He thought if I took on sole responsibility for her welfare it would impact adversely on my life. I explained to him that I was in a position to do this, having few other responsibilities. Plus, with the nursing home up for sale, I'd struggle to find alternative accommodation for her because of the high levels of noise she was capable of generating.

He agreed to help. Dr A rang the re-ablement services while I was there, to arrange for them to visit the home to assess Joan's care needs. After that had been done, he'd call another meeting to discuss my mother's requirements and whether I could meet them. I had to wait to hear from Dr A.

Towards the end of November I heard from Louise that Registration had received a complaint about Katrina and they were now gunning for her. Not before time. Everyone who was working their notice had been asked to make a statement about her. Louise thought that I was the one who'd made the complaint. Sadly, I had to disillusion her.

By mid-December, Katrina had been suspended and Brian was refusing to talk to anyone who'd been prepared to make a statement.

A visit to my mother in December 2000 typified the dire situation she was now in. Mum was in her room and shouting, barely pausing to draw breath. Her left eye was glued shut, now almost a permanent condition. A thigh strap was being used again to secure her catheter bag to her calf, wound round her leg twice, and the bag was full. Obviously it was still leaking as her trousers and chair were both wet, which meant that she was in a worse position than before. I could see no valid reason for this invasive procedure.

I questioned Brian about the efficacy of catheterisation. He admitted that Joan had a new catheter put in the day before as the previous one had blocked up after only two weeks when it should've lasted for two months.

I drew his attention to my mother's sorry plight. His response was weary silence. No mention from him that both her proposed key worker and care worker were leaving, neither did he query the reason for the visit by the re-ablement representative who'd been to assess Mum. When I left, she still hadn't been changed, although I'd emptied the catheter bag before I went.

A week before Christmas, I had a phone call from Brian to tell me that Joan was unwell with a chest infection. The doctor had started her on antibiotics, but they would probably be putting her on a subcutaneous drip as they hadn't been able to persuade her to take sufficient food or fluids and were afraid that the catheter would block up.

I waited until 11pm then phoned Louise, who was on night duty. Louise said that Joan had been asleep since she'd started work, but she didn't think that my mother was experiencing any breathing problems. She said that Joan was on a drip as they'd only managed to get 700ml of fluid into her during the day. For the sake of the catheter, she needed more.

The next day I went to see Mum. Although she was asleep, there was no evidence of a chest infection, her breathing and pulse rate were good and steady and she'd been shouting earlier in the day. The nurse on duty, Rachel, said that her blood pressure was low and they'd sent off a urine specimen to check for a UTI. She also told me that Joan had been re-catheterised again. Brian had neglected to tell me that.

The drip had been discontinued and Mum drank a beaker of cordial when she woke up, but it took a while. I noticed that the catheter bag was lying beside her in the bed, instead of being fixed to a stand below her hips. There was never any evidence of a stand in her bedroom, so I surmised that this may have been the normal practice, but such bad practice. My guess was there was no chest infection as yet and Mum was far more likely to have a UTI again.

That night I mentally drafted yet another letter to Brian.

The draft made it into print on the third day. He needed to know that I was more cognisant about unfolding events at HM than he probably realised.

I told him that I understood that both Louise and Vicky, proposed key worker and care worker respectively, were leaving at the end of the month. I'd been waiting to hear from him in relation to this, as the end of December was looming fast.

I appreciated that he wasn't able to stop staff leaving but normally there wasn't a great deal of movement with workers anywhere this close to Christmas, so this was an indicator of a disgruntled workforce. He also needed to know that information about Mum would be better coming from him, than leaked to me by a significant number of moles within his domain.

I'm also concerned about Joan's catheterisation, I wrote. *I understand that she has now been re-catheterised twice since the original one was inserted. As you know, I had misgivings about this invasive procedure from the outset and I haven't had my fears allayed, in any way, so far.*

I've had very little feedback from you about this situation, but if you think that catheterisation is still a good idea, please sell it to me, because at the moment I'm unconvinced and feel that, for my mother, there is no advantage to this procedure.

I was working over Christmas that year so fitted in a visit with Bob on the 22nd December. Mum was much improved and shouting. She'd had a bath that morning and was sitting with wet hair, normal practice it seemed. Nobody saw the need to dry hair with a hairdryer.

Two care assistants came into the room to check that Joan had been given her 10am cup of tea (it was then 11am). They knew that neither of them had given it to her and presumed that, as the cup had gone, somebody else must have done it.

I'd observed before that kitchen staff come round and collect cups from the rooms after a reasonable length of time. They had very likely removed what would've been a cold and undrinkable cup of tea.

Mum wasn't in a reclined position, apparently Brian doesn't approve of her being reclined because her legs are then up and the urine drains backwards. The problem being, that the reclined position prevented her from continually sliding out of the chair and onto the floor.

If she had to sit upright, then that wasn't a suitable chair for her, because her feet didn't touch the ground and there was subsequently too much pressure on the back of her thighs. Everything, it seemed, was geared around making catheterisation work, which it obviously wasn't. My mother's overall comfort was low priority. If Brian was insisting on this, then she should have been in her other armchair, which was lower.

I was about to relay my thoughts to Bob, when I noticed that Mum's catheter bag was very low down on her leg again, visible below her trouser leg. On investigation it was obvious that it wasn't strapped at all. In her upright position, the weight of the bag of urine was hanging from her bladder, unsupported.

I began to tremble with anger, Bob stood up to go and find Brian. I called him back, because we both needed to calm down. The staff already knew that I wanted to see him, to give him the letter.

Brian came into Mum's room shortly after my discovery. I showed him the problem and he started to spout all the excuses that we'd heard before. This was too much for Bob, who usually lets me do the talking. He's not by nature a fast mover, but the speed with which he left his chair and parked himself within Brian's personal space was motivated by fury. Bob squared up to the manager, his jaw jutted forward. I could see that Brian was rattled.

'I don't want to hear any more excuses or listen to you blaming everybody else. What we want is the immediate problem sorted now and proper care given to my mother, starting today!' Bob said.

I hadn't intended talking to Registration until after Joan was out of HM, but I wondered if I could afford to wait, not that I had much faith in their motivation to take action.

Chapter Fifteen

It was a turning point. I'd planned to move Mum out of the nursing home, but to be honest, I hadn't done much about it in a practical sense. I needed to focus on the next steps to turn this into a fact rather than whimsy. I resolved to start looking for the right property, in the right place, at the right price. I would decide what equipment I was going to need, source suppliers and draft a rough outline of the initial setup and financial outlay.

The other vital ingredient was finding somebody I trusted to work as a carer for my mother for the times I needed to be off duty. I already had somebody in mind, but would she be interested?

Jodi was a night care worker and we often worked together. With just two care assistants in the same bungalow for ten hours, we'd got to know each other pretty well. I always enjoyed working with Jodi, she was easy, open and didn't flap or panic. She carried out the work she had to do efficiently and had a quiet, confident way with the residents, who trusted and accepted her and were happy to cooperate. This, I'm sorry to say, wasn't the case with all the staff.

There was one girl I dreaded working with. She was quite an introverted little soul, which made it a long night. Her timidity was felt by some of the more discerning residents, who reacted adversely to her obvious lack of confidence.

The problem, as I saw it, was that this was a different client group for her. Snow White (if you'd seen her, you'd know why she'd acquired that name in my head) had been used to working with the elderly in a residential home. I could imagine she would have won minds and hearts in that role. Working with adults who had severe learning disabilities is a whole different ball game, sweet and demure just won't cut it. She was being eaten alive.

I tried to help, but it got lost in translation and made matters worse instead of better. She reported me to the manager for undermining her. I apologised of course, though I was never clear what I was apologising for, but for the sake of peace, I backed off. I know I can be a little acerbic at times, I'm an acquired taste perhaps, but hey, I've got enough of my own insecurities to keep a psychiatric team in full employment. I decided I couldn't handle somebody else's, so I let her get on with it without interference.

Snow White continued to work with the residents although she had no idea how to interact with them. I had to bite my tongue and try to ignore the resulting mayhem, as she got chewed up and spat out. I grudgingly admired her, because she kept coming back for more, but always with the same result. Fortunately, I didn't have to work with her too often, and we did develop a workable relationship, which no doubt required equal effort on both sides.

Jodi was my kind of care worker. She worked two nights a week which was convenient because she had a small daughter, not yet at school. Her partner worked full-time, but there wasn't enough money coming in.

I ran it past her, hypothetically. I didn't know how many hours exactly, but it would be at least twelve hours a week at the same hourly rate she was getting then and she could bring her little girl with her. The downside was that the hours would be fragmented and I couldn't guarantee how long the job would last for. Jodi was unnervingly animated about it all, especially as I didn't feel anywhere close to making the job I was describing into a reality.

In the wee small hours, we discussed the shortcomings of Huesneath Moor nursing home and came to the conclusion that we could make a better job of it, even without nursing qualifications and a uniform. Now, suddenly it all seemed possible. We left it that Jodi would have first option on the vacancy.

***

When I visited HM on Boxing Day, Katrina immediately came fussing around (unfortunately, she'd been reinstated). I'd had this "Uriah Heep" treatment before, after a set-to with staff.

'Will it be alright if I book Joan in with the hairdresser?' she asked.

'I don't usually get consulted, it's understood that she should have her hair cut whenever it's deemed necessary,' I replied. 'Oh, and can she be booked in for a manicure at the same time? Her nails are excessively long.'

Katrina said she would ask a care assistant to cut them that day.

While I was there, Mum gradually slid down the chair until her back was more on the seat than her bum and I had to ask for help to get her sitting upright again. She needed to be in a reclined position otherwise she would end up on the floor. This was a concept that even an amoeba could get its cell around.

If I'd harboured the desire that maybe Huesneath Moor would start the new year with positive resolutions, I would have been sorely disappointed. Bob came with me on the first visit of 2001. It was easier to visit together when we could, the hate vibes from some of the staff were becoming palpable and we certainly didn't feel like welcome visitors. Mum was in her room, in a reclined position, but very wet. I didn't notice until after she'd been changed that she no longer had a catheter in.

Brian was on duty, but he didn't mention anything about the catheter, my letter, or the key worker scheme. Mum's nails had been cut, but in doing so they'd damaged one finger, causing a blood blister and bleeding under the fingernail.

A cup of tea was brought in at about 3pm with some sponge cake mashed up in milk.

'Joan is quite capable of eating a piece of sponge cake in its original form, though I appreciate that it does take longer to feed her with it.' I said.

The care assistant started to get defensive and then thought better of it, turned on her heels and disappeared, returning with a recognisable piece of cake.

I didn't know if they'd conceded defeat over the catheter or if it had blocked up again and there had been no alternative but to remove it. Maybe, Mum had ended up on the floor so many times from her upright sitting position that even they could see it wasn't going to work. To be honest, I was too tired for another confrontation.

***

On the way home Bob and I discussed the progress of our plan to spring Mum out of HM. I told him that now the extended closure of businesses during Christmas and the New Year was over, I'd begin the search for a suitable bungalow in earnest. I had a list of things to do.

I had one small niggle over all this.

'What happens if we get all this together and Mum dies without ever leaving that place? We'll have bought property and equipped it with her money.'

Bob looked at me with that expression on his face which told me that he thought I was a complete idiot.

'Then we'll be the owners of a bungalow in Bideford. It won't be a problem. But don't do anything about selling your place until we've secured a bungalow for Mum, just in case this doesn't work out.'

It sounded so simple coming from him.

***

Armed with bungalow details, I trawled the streets of Bideford, Northam and Westward Ho! I left Appledore out of the equation, the house prices there were always inflated and it had hills.

I don't tend to do hills, I'll always try to walk round them. I lived at the top of Bideford while Jake was at the pushchair age. With no car, it was a tidy old walk to where the action was, Victoria Park, the River Torridge and the shops, but it was all downhill. Coming back, however, was another story. The steepest hill is Bridge Street and pushing a chunky toddler up that road was a recipe for a cardiac arrest. After surviving that free test for the condition of the heart, I continued uphill, all the way home.

House viewing always makes me feel uncomfortable and fraudulent. I feel compelled to explain the circumstances, lest the home owners think I'm a time waster, just brightening up my drab life gawping at other people's décor. Then there is the need to be complimentary, even if the place is crammed to the gunnels with hoarded tat and smells of cat's pee.

In fairness, all the places I viewed were presentable, but I had a specific agenda, which was more to do with a workable layout than designer wallpaper.

The place needed to have three bedrooms. The third room, even if it was only a box room, would be required if I got sick and needed to employ care staff on a twenty-four hour basis for an extended period. Sometimes it's easier to find somebody who's prepared to live in for a short while. I had a friend who did that for a living. She shared the 24/7 care with another woman and worked two weeks on, living in, and two weeks off, in her own home. It was an arrangement that worked well for the two of them. The clients, an elderly married couple, had the added bonus of continuity of care and being able to build a relationship with their care workers.

So, three bedrooms were a must, plus a garden requiring minimum maintenance with wheelchair accessibility. The bungalow needed to have an uncomplicated room layout with hallways wide enough for a wheelchair and a hoist. The bathroom had to be big enough to put the hoist next to the bath to transfer Mum to a bath chair, which would then lift and swivel and be lowered into the water. I also wanted flat access to the place, no hill, no steps, no hassle.

I didn't think there would be a problem finding properties that met my criteria but there weren't a vast number that ticked many, if any, of the boxes. Having thrown away the details of the definitely unacceptable, I was left with six to view and out of those, only two were worth a second look.

One was at Westward Ho! and the land couldn't have been flatter. The estate was built on ground reclaimed from the sea and although the properties had been there for a good number of years, I'd always viewed it as a likely casualty if global warming ever took off in Westward Ho! As it was, Northam Burrows, which lay between the housing estate and the sea separated only by a road, was a sodden bog throughout the winter. Then I was told by somebody with inside knowledge that the properties in that particular part of the estate had ongoing drainage problems that could prove costly to rectify.

That left a bungalow in Bideford, not exactly on flat land, as it was at the top of the town. The estate itself though, was fairly level and I didn't envisage pushing a wheelchair into town and back. Mum wasn't nearly well enough to undergo trips out and about.

***

The couple who lived there wanted to move back to Luton to be near the assistance of their family. The husband had suffered a severe stroke which had left him paralysed on one side of his body. His intellect appeared unaffected, but his speech was slow and slurred and required time to tune into, making communication difficult and frustrating for both him and his listeners. I heard from the next door neighbours that he'd been a belligerent old devil when he'd been well. He'd ruled his wife like a regimental sergeant major and was always warring verbally with neighbours over trifling issues. No wonder he'd had a stroke, his blood pressure must have been permanently sky high.

The bungalow was dated and it was obvious that imaginative décor hadn't been his forte, but the layout filled my requirements. His wife was obviously coping with pushing a wheelchair around the place. It had three bedrooms and the kitchen was a long galley style room that led, through a greenhouse/conservatory affair, into the garden, all on the level. The garden was a disaster. It'd been on the receiving end of nil maintenance for a considerable period of time.

Apparently, the space had been used as an allotment to grow fruit and vegetables. The only garden, as such, had been a patch of grass in one corner about four feet square, where his wife was permitted to sit in a deckchair.

I was quietly horrified. To turn this bit of ground which had reverted to field grass and brambles into an easily maintained garden would be a challenge. If I took it on, it would be time and energy consuming and to have it done professionally would be prohibitively expensive. Still, given that this was the only place that, in all other respects, was suitable, was I being a too picky about the garden? I could wait for the perfect place to come onto the market, but realistically, was that likely?

I rang Bob, who passed the ball back into my court. I was, after all, the best judge on what was required. He didn't think that the garden should be a deal breaker, because it was rectifiable. He arranged for a surveyor to give it the once over. His pronouncement was favourable. A little dated, a touch of rot in the window ledge at the front of the place, but a sound, if unremarkable property.

Bob put in an offer just below the asking price to reflect the work that would be needed to create a garden. I didn't think the owner, Mr Grumpy, would be too keen on an offer of less than the asking price, but I was hoping his family would want to get things moving. They'd already found a property in Luton and needed the funds to secure it.

We were using a local solicitor for the purchase of the bungalow simply because I knew one of the conveyance clerks. We were also involved with a firm of solicitors recommended by the Alzheimer's Society, because we had nagging doubts about Social Services' refusal to be involved in what we were about to do. We had an initial meeting with Miss Gray, one of the solicitors. She'd shaken her head in disbelief as I relayed the telephone conversations I'd had with Social Services. Miss Gray explained that they'd have to be involved at some point, whether they wanted to be or not. I guess that's what I was afraid of, that we'd get so far down the road, buying a bungalow, handing in my notice at work and so forth, then Social Services would wake up and say, 'No, you can't do this.'

***

When I arrived to visit Mum during the first week of January, I found she 'd been put to bed. My mother was unwell with a heavy cold. Katrina told me that they were waiting for antibiotics for a suspected UTI and a chest infection. She passed urine while I was there and it was certainly offensive. I tried to give her a cup of tea, but she wouldn't take it, though Katrina managed to get a full beaker of squash down her, just before I left.

Mum was certainly full of phlegm, which, although it sounded loose enough, she couldn't expel. I doubted whether she actually had a chest infection — yet. Katrina said she'd become unwell with this cold a day or two after my last visit.

I thought, under the circumstances, I should've been informed. Mum wasn't eating, but they were giving her a food supplement drink. There was, I thought, cause for concern, as she was in a debilitated state to begin with.

The catheter hadn't been replaced and Katrina said that as far as she knew they weren't going to re-catheterise as it was continually blocking up. Joan was obviously not a suitable candidate.

I rang HM at 2pm the next day to find out if there was any improvement in my mother's condition. I spoke to the owner, Mr B who didn't know anything about it and went to find somebody who did. The reply he gave me was that she had a suspected urinary tract infection and was very sleepy. I replied that I'd been in to visit her the day before and really wanted to know if her condition had improved, or not, since then. He said he couldn't tell me as he hadn't seen her, but if I wanted, he would ask Brian to ring me. As I was unable to believe one word that man said, I declined his offer rather ungraciously.

When I visited in the morning two days later, Mum was sitting in her chair. Her room was equally as freezing as the cup of tea on her bedside table, which nobody had bothered to give her. She was full of cold, both eyes glued shut with yellow gunk and both nostrils blocked with hardened mucus. She was wearing a thin, long sleeved vest and a cardigan, that wasn't hers.

I bathed her eyes clear of muck with cotton wool and was in the process of de-coking her nose, when Katrina came into the room. She informed me that, although she'd told me three days ago that Joan would be receiving antibiotics for her UTI, it hadn't happened yet. They couldn't get a sample of urine from her.

I suppressed the volcano threatening to erupt from within, as I pointed out to Katrina exactly what I was doing and why. I think she could sense that I wasn't best pleased.

'I know you won't believe me, but I was just about to do those jobs,' she said.

I asked for some cotton buds and Vaseline so that I could coat the inside of Mum's nostrils to make her nose less sore and easier to clean. I also asked for a decongestant to help her breath a little easier.

Katrina returned with cotton buds and baby oil (useless) and no decongestant. Because these were over the counter preparations and not on prescription, I'd have to provide them for Joan, she told me. How the volcano didn't register on the Volcanic Explosivity Index as I attempted to swallow down my anger, I'm not sure.

Katrina also suggested that as antibiotics were not going to be available until at least Wednesday when Dr A did his rounds, (although it was obvious to anyone with a sense of smell that my mother had another UTI) perhaps I should buy some cranberry juice for her.

Now, while I had no objection to buying anything that my mother needed, surely things like decongestants should've been in the home's general supplies, along with plasters and antiseptic? The clue was in the name — nursing home. Even a reverse charge telephone call to ask me to bring these items in would have been preferable to doing absolutely nothing.

When I returned from my shopping expedition for nursing supplies, Mum was being washed and changed out of her inappropriate clothing. Some idiot had given her a throat sweet to suck. An ideal piece of hard candy for a woman who was deemed unable to eat a slice of cake unless it's dissolved in milk. The sweet inevitably made her cough and choke and she was violently sick, all down the cardigan that wasn't hers. As it happened, it was no bad thing, because she threw up a vast quantity of mucus and subsequently ate a good lunch.

***

I had an appointment to see Dr A. Neither he nor I had heard anything from Social Services although the solicitor had written informing them that under some Act or another, they were obliged to be an active participant. I couldn't say I really wanted them to be an active participant now. I had the feeling that it wasn't going to work to our advantage, because nobody likes to be told that they've got it wrong.

I'd prepared a detailed Care Plan for Dr A's perusal. I must admit, a lot of it was based on my general experience rather than tailored to my mother's needs, because apart from observation, I knew very few details about my mother's condition. The nursing home had never been strong on keeping me in the loop. But as Care Plans went, it was as good as any that I'd read and I'd read quite a few.

It was a joint effort between Kathy, the care worker I'd been on duty with a couple of nights before, and me. She was thinking about doing a similar thing for her mother who'd suffered a devastating stroke and was now in a hospital, receiving care that Kathy classed as inadequate at best, barbaric at worst. She spent most of her off duty time there and felt she could do a far better job than the hospital was doing. I believed her.

I left a copy of the Care Plan at the surgery so that Dr A would have an opportunity to look through it before our meeting scheduled for the 12th January.

Chapter Sixteen

CARE PLAN

WAKING UP/WASHING/GROOMING

Joan is often more relaxed and amenable first thing in the morning. She can be blanket-bathed on the bed or transferred, using hoist and wheelchair, to the bathroom and bathed. If Joan has been incontinent of faeces, I would clean her up on the bed and then bath her.

Joan requires a bath at least three times a week. Her hair gets greasy quickly and it's easier to wash her hair in the bath. Joan's ears get a frequent build up of wax in the outer ear. I need to ensure that they're kept clean otherwise this will be a source of irritation. Her eyes are invariably glued shut in the mornings, this has been an ongoing problem for some while and there is a need to bathe her eyes every morning, possibly using a weak saline solution.

Her finger and toe nails need to be kept short and clean. I would keep Joan's hair trimmed myself, as it will be easier to do when she is in a quiet, content mood.

Check daily for any skin problems, e.g. reddening or breaks in the skin to pressure areas and urine burn to the groin. I personally like a barrier/cleansing cream for general use and that seems to work well in the prevention and treatment of urine burn.

DRESSING

Joan is resistant to carers moving her limbs, so stretchy, loose fitting, front fastening clothes are more appropriate. Trousers are better than skirts for warmth and personal dignity, as her legs are often drawn up. Her feet are usually cold so socks and slippers are suitable for indoor use and fleecy lined boots if she's outside. Joan loses body heat very quickly as her mobility is limited and her body fat virtually non existent.

MOBILITY

Very limited mobility. On the Norton Scale, a process for the assessment of pressure ulcer risk, she scores as being at high risk of developing sores. Joan cannot walk or weight bear. She has a fair range of movement in her legs, however, but not in her upper body, head and arms, which are tense with a limited range of movement. Joan will slide down from a sitting position on a chair and onto the floor so a lap and possibly a groin belt will be required in a wheelchair. Use of a recliner helps to keep her in the chair without restricting her other movements, it also allows Joan to move her legs freely without any pressure to the back of the thighs. At present her skin condition is good.

MEALS

Joan's false teeth went missing about eighteen months ago because she kept taking them out. At present she has a good appetite and eats and drinks well. Her food has to be soft, mashed or liquidised though she can, at present, manage some textures, e.g. sponge cake, crustless sandwiches with a soft filling, cut into small squares.

A nutritionally good diet and plenty of clear fluids, in addition to hot beverages, are essential to maintain her physical well being for as long as possible, but she has developed a sweet tooth as the dementia has progressed and at this stage, I certainly do not intend to deprive her of the treats she enjoys.

TOILETING

Joan is doubly incontinent. She has proved not to be a suitable candidate for catheterisation. Joan has to wear pads and I favour the nappy type Tena slip pads that fix at the front with adhesive tapes. At present, Joan wears shaped pads but manages to urinate around them because they are difficult to position correctly. At present Joan doesn't wear a pad at night. There are arguments for and against this practice, but personally I'm in favour of padding at night.

I understand that Joan takes daily medication to help move her bowel and as a rule is able to evacuate her bowel unaided, usually in the morning, after breakfast, so that would be a good time to use the commode. She does occasionally become constipated and sometimes when she is noisy, this will be the reason. It will be necessary therefore to keep a record of bowel movements.

LIFTING AND HANDLING

Joan is a slightly built woman who is unable to walk or bear her own weight. There is also rigidity in her body and limbs and resistance to being moved. A hoist will be required to transfer Joan between bed, wheelchair, recliner, commode and bath. Ideally, I would like to have the use of a net sling for the bath, a toilet sling and a transfer sling. I will need to be able to bath her at home and for this I will require a chair that can be fixed to the bath, which can then be swung outside the bath, to allow for transfer and be raised and lowered. I will also require a transfer board to move Joan from wheelchair to car seat.

BEDTIME

Going to bed would be a reversal of the morning regimen. The bed would need to be a hospital type bed as procedures such as washing and dressing will take place on the bed and a domestic type will be too low. The bed would require a waterproof mattress and incontinence bed pads with tuck in flaps will be acquired, to be used over the bottom sheet.

She prefers her left side for sleeping but obviously must have a change of position but, as yet, I don't know how mobile Joan is when in bed. Presuming that she can move herself onto her back, I would think that a four-hourly check would be sufficient. This will ensure that Joan is not wet or soiled and that her position in bed is altered, to minimize the risk of pressure sores developing. I appreciate that this will have to be reviewed as her condition deteriorates further. It may necessitate buying in some night care at a future date. I also think that a baby monitor between rooms might be required.

DAYTIME ACTIVITIES

The nature of dementia sufferers means that changes of environment are often upsetting and stimulation is not always welcomed. Joan's quality of life, due to her illness, is very impoverished but, at present, there are flashes of awareness still and times when there is social interaction, albeit at a very basic level.

Joan's degree of alertness has actually improved since being removed from the isolation of her room and placed in the lounge for a couple of hours during the morning. To me it indicates that she still welcomes variety and being part of a social group. I hope to include the outdoors into her environment via the garden and even short trips out in her wheelchair. Obviously, I'll have to see if that distresses her or not. Joan will certainly be getting more company, on a one to one basis and through the coming and going of family and friends.

Joan appears to pay no attention to the television, but since her glasses went missing eighteen months ago, I doubt if she can actually see the television screen. Music may well provide an alternative that can be appreciated at some level. Massage is another very beneficial therapy for many reasons and I know she used to enjoy having her feet massaged so I'll explore this avenue with her.

COMMUNICATION

Joan has no meaningful verbal communication. Very occasionally she'll say an isolated word and sometimes this is said in the appropriate place, but this is rare. Joan shouts a lot, especially during the afternoons. The reasons for her shouting are not always discernible but sometimes there is actually, or coincidentally, a reason for this, e.g. soiled, wet, thirsty, hungry, anxiety at being moved, etc. Empathy is required to try to minimise the obvious causes for this behaviour.

SENSORY DIFFICULTIES

Joan lost her glasses about eighteen months ago. She's very short sighted so her vision beyond a limited range will be indistinct. To test her eyesight would now be impossible, so the reintroduction of glasses, after this time lapse, would not be feasible.

Joan lost her false teeth about eighteen months ago and fitting her for new dentures would not really be possible after this time lapse. It does mean that she loses the pleasure of different textures, so it's important that, although her food has to be mashed or liquidised, it is presented in such a way that she can appreciate individual flavours.

BEHAVIOURAL TENDENCIES

Joan was admitted to Huesneath Moor from a residential home because she had become very agitated and physically aggressive. I'm informed that she's on a cocktail of three different drugs from the tranquiliser, anti-psychotic and anti-anxiety genre, which were prescribed to keep her relatively calm. Joan dislikes being moved or manhandled and resists, verbally and physically. She has very noisy spells, shouting at top volume. There maybe a reason for this, but that reason is not always discernible. There are still occasional glimpses of her sense of humour. Something, somebody says or does will start her laughing and sometimes she will pull a comical face to, it would seem, amuse others or express her own feelings.

MEDICAL MATTERS

Joan has been prescribed three different drugs to reduce her levels of agitation and aggression. I haven't been informed which drugs she's taking, although I know that she still takes paroxetine and that she's also given Lorazepam. Joan also receives medication to avoid constipation.

Joan is doubly incontinent and has proved not to be a suitable candidate for catheterisation. She has frequent urine infections so it is essential that fluid levels are kept high.

Joan has haemorrhoids which occasionally require treatment with appropriate cream and apparently the use of witch hazel which, her key worker informs me, is very effective.

Joan sometimes suffers with constipation which requires an enema. A bowel chart would be a good idea just to ensure that she doesn't remain impacted. This is another good reason why fluid intake levels should be kept high.

FAMILY CONTACT

My brother visits Joan at HM about four times a month and these visits would continue, probably more frequently, once she is home. My son has only visited his Gran two or three times since her move to HM, but would be a frequent visitor at home. Joan has three surviving siblings, living in Birmingham, one of whom would visit from time to time.

RISK ASSESSMENT

This is a degenerative condition and although the rate of deterioration appears to have slowed, I think that's largely because Joan's faculties are now so impoverished that deterioration isn't so obvious.

She requires twenty-four hour care but, at present, a fair percentage of that is the necessity to have somebody always there because she's vulnerable. As her condition deteriorates, the amount of physical care required will inevitably increase. Feeding may become a problem if her ability to swallow becomes impaired. Her skin viability will also possibly become more difficult to maintain.

Joan will probably withdraw more into herself and flashes of response will become negligible or non existent.

I'll need to keep in mind the possibility that Joan will need an increased level of outside care. I've based her present care needs on twelve to fifteen hours of purchased care per week, in addition to the care she will receive from me. This may well increase, especially if night care becomes necessary. I will require break periods for myself and anticipate that four weeks of respite care will be required, spaced throughout the year. This may present a problem as there are not many nursing homes that are happy about taking on somebody as noisy as Joan. Full-time care in the home is prohibitively expensive and would necessitate me going away to get a proper break, which I won't necessarily want to do.

There is also the possibility that I may get ill and be unable to care for Joan myself. If that should happen, then my brother and I would have to re-assess the possibility of buying in twenty-four hour care or respite care, if it was a short term illness, or re-admitting Joan into a nursing home, that is best suited to her needs at that time.

OVERVIEW

Given my age and state of health and my mother's state of health at the present time, I'm certain that I can give her better physical care than she is receiving now and provide Joan with an enhanced quality of life. I also feel that I can meet her immediate needs and will be able to continue to meet those needs throughout the foreseeable deterioration in her condition that is symptomatic of dementia of the Alzheimer's type.

Chapter Seventeen

12th February, 2001 - Meeting with Dr A, Grace (re-ablement team), Trish (Abbotsvale). Social Services were unable to attend.

Dr A said that he was very doubtful that care levels were likely to improve at HM. He'd explored the possibility of moving Joan to another nursing home and had to agree with my findings. Joan's noisy episodes and the fact that she had been assessed as EMI made it unlikely that any good nursing home would want to take her on a long term basis. Trish suggested the other EMI unit, the one I'd visited prior to choosing Joan's present accommodation. I wouldn't entertain the idea.

Trish was concerned that the noise levels Joan was capable of generating would prove too much for me to cope with. She likened it to the stress caused to a single mum, with a baby that constantly cries. I knew she was thinking about the episode when I assaulted Joan which was the reason why she had to go into a care home in the first place. I had no concrete answers, except to explain that I was in a different place, mentally, since choosing to live apart from my husband, and I didn't see Joan as my mother any more. I no longer had unreasonable expectations that she should, somehow, still fulfil that role. I was effectively adopting a baby, who would continue to grow down instead of up. Trish didn't say any more, but I could tell by her body language that she was far from convinced that I was going to be able to cope with Joan at home.

Grace had assessed Joan at HM and didn't think that the re-ablement unit could offer anything, as she had deteriorated too far. She had, however, got an agreement from Social Services that they would appoint a care manager for Joan, as they had a duty of care. In view of that, she was disappointed that Social Services had been unable to attend.

Dr A felt that Joan was too poorly to be moved at the moment, having had two bouts of pneumonia and septicaemia, all within the last month. (Needless to say the home hadn't informed me of the seriousness of her condition.) But having read my care plan, he was in agreement that I could take her into my care if, or when, Joan became well enough to be moved.

I went to see Mum that afternoon. She still sounded full of cold, but was very alert and vastly improved from two days before.

***

Three days after the meeting with Dr A, I had an appointment to see my GP who'd also been Mum's before she went into Huesneath Moor. I wanted him to be her doctor again, when I took over as carer. I needed to see him to

106

ascertain how he felt about it. Would he be as disquieted as Trish obviously was? He was the one who had to pick up the pieces when I turned up at his surgery, distraught because I'd assaulted my mother. I'd rather hear his opinion at the outset.

He couldn't have been sweeter.

'Of course I'll be Joan's doctor. She was my first patient when I came to the Bideford surgery as a GP so she's special to me.'

He said he was happy to give my mother and me all the support he could.

'You're going to do a brilliant job,' he said.

I felt elated. He'd said all the right things, nothing negative, all positive, and I left feeling that I could take on the world.

The surgery, hospital and Social Services were all within close proximity of each other, so I called into the hospital to see what equipment I'd be able to acquire from them.

The re-ablement team was based at the hospital so I took the liberty of popping in, on the off chance that Grace was around. She very kindly explained how equipment was accessed. It was a mishmash, the Health Authority providing some equipment and Social Services providing other bits of kit like the wheelchair and hoist. I could order incontinence pads through the local Health Authority who delivered to the door in bulk. I just had to let them know what type and how many for the month.

The hospital would lend me a hospital bed, providing there was one available, but they were in short supply. At that time, all the beds were out on loan, so we may have to buy our own. Grace said she would pull a few strings and try to get Joan a pressure relieving airwave mattress. This type is ribbed and has air pumping through the mattress in a continuous wave motion, throughout its length. It would mean that I wouldn't have to turn Mum so frequently through the night. I'd got this item on my list, but it would be brilliant if we could have one on loan.

I was on a roll, so decided to visit Social Services to find out how to access their cache of equipment. I'd heard nothing from them, and time was of the essence now, as the offer Bob had made on the bungalow had been accepted. I attempted to explain to the receptionist why I was there, why I had no appointment and why I had no idea who I was supposed to make an appointment with. She asked me to take a seat. I couldn't hear the telephone conversation that took place, except to say it was lengthy.

I didn't know the man walking towards me, but if I had to guess, by the insincere smile, I would have said Mr Jones, and so it proved to be. I was escorted to his office. I'd like to report that he was apologetic. It's difficult to hold a grudge against somebody who says, 'I'm sorry, I got it wrong.'

Our face to face meeting was no more successful than our telephone conversation in November. Having been, I suspected, humiliated into playing an active part in this, he now realised that the telephone conversation we had was inappropriate. He had the gall to re-invent the entire conversation and the audacity to try it out on me, I guess to see if I would accept his revised version of events.

If he'd been in touch with me prior to that day, or had sent a representative to the meeting, I'd probably have let it go. But as things stood, I protested vehemently and reminded him how the conversation had actually gone. Not one of my better moves, if you need to get people on your side. His response was to tell me that it was his word against mine. I had to admit that he had the upper hand.

My brother later pointed out, when I related the event to him, that we'd no reason to lie about the conversation that took place. We'd been the ones to initiate all the right moves to comply with the correct procedures, whereas he'd got every reason to fabricate the contents of that phone call because the truth made him look like an incompetent prat. If Mr Jones hadn't got me so totally rattled, I'd have had great pleasure in telling the incompetent prat just that. Fortunately, the original telephone conversation had been relayed verbally by me, to Dr A and Miss Gray, the solicitor, just after the event.

I came away with my high spirit brought low again, but I'd secured an appointment with the social worker who would be Mum's care manager.

***

I gave up making diary entries at this point. Events were moving fast and I didn't have the time, anyway it was obvious that HM was never going to change, not on Brian's watch at any rate. It would need Registration's boot up their backside before there would be any possibility of improvement.

I'd arranged the appointment with the Social Services' care manager appointed to Mum at a time when Bob would be available to come with me. In view of past dealings with Mr Jones, I wanted my brother's ears and brain in case things got nasty.

It transpired that the care manager, Sandra, appeared to be in total ignorance about the events that had led up to this meeting. My brother enlightened her and brought her up to speed. As a union representative, he had a way with words that always sounded very authoritative.

He explained that Social Services had, up to this point, refused any involvement. But, because they'd been made aware of their duty of care, initially by his sister (me) then by Mum's GP, our solicitor and the re-ablement team, Social Services now, at the eleventh hour, realised that they needed to be seen to have input and potentially had the power to scupper the whole plan. Bob's veiled point was that, if that happened, he would go public.

He stressed that the notes and diary that I'd been keeping, with reference to the abuse our mother was being subjected to on a daily basis, would be sent to Registration as soon as Mum had been removed. The only reason a complaint hadn't been made official before now, was fear of reprisals while she was still in their care.

Give Sandra her due, she managed to maintain a sympathetic and concerned attitude, without actually acknowledging any fault on behalf of Social Services. Of course, she may have been accustomed to accusations being levelled at her boss and had learnt how to field them.

At the end of the meeting, we came away with nothing, except the realisation that we had to wait for Social Services to say yes or no. Not at all satisfactory, but our hands were tied.

Bob reckoned that it was just red tape. They'd have to say yes or come up with some very good reasons why we couldn't. As it stood, both GPs had already agreed to it, the solicitor recommended by the Alzheimer's Society was on our side and HM was up for sale. Bob didn't think there was much to worry about. I sincerely hoped he was right. My cottage had been on the market for only two weeks and the first person who'd viewed it had made an offer of virtually the full asking price.

***

I'd done some rough calculations, and Bob had given them the once over. I wanted fifteen to twenty hours of purchased care a week. I'd sourced local suppliers for nearly all the special equipment we'd need except her commode and adjustable bedside table which were at the nursing home. Bed, airwave mattress, wheelchair, hoist and adjustable seat for the bath were, I hoped, being provided by the local Health Authority or Social Services.

I'd dropped a note through Jodi's door, giving her a typical week's duty roster. Some of the duties would be fixed to cover my meetings at the Kingdom Hall, which accounted for about eight hours, the remainder was more or less negotiable. My guesstimate was mid-March before everything was in place, so it would give Jodi time to think it through. I knew money was tight, and if she could possibly do it, she would.

Bob was happy with the cost of it all. Even taking into account the lump sum used to purchase the bungalow. There was still enough money coming in through pensions, carer's allowance, attendance allowance and interest on investments to fund it all. Interest rates were still good in February of 2001. My father had received a healthy occupational pension, a good percentage of which had passed to my mother when he died. It was going to be okay. I repeated the phrase like a mantra, often said with more hope than conviction.

Jodi said yes. The only problem was Sundays. Her partner hadn't been happy about a regular Sunday duty. I could see his point, he worked full-time and was still playing in a band and had a regular Saturday night gig. Sundays were for recovery and family. My Sunday meetings were set in stone as far as I was concerned so, rather than risk losing Jodi, I decided to employ somebody just for the Sunday duty. It would only be for a couple of hours, but surely someone suitable would step up to the plate?

Jodi said she'd be happy to start off doing the Sundays until I found a replacement. She reasoned as my meeting was in the morning and her partner slept until midday, he wasn't going to miss her until lunchtime. That was fine as a temporary measure, but because two congregations shared the hall, the meeting time would change to the afternoon next year, so I definitely had to find another carer, but the pressure was off for the moment.

***

Everything was falling into place, I'd accepted the offer on my cottage, the purchase of the bungalow was at the exchange of contract stage and I was working my month's notice at the residential home. We were still waiting on Social Services and I was sick to death of metaphorically holding my breath. It seemed grossly unreasonable that Social Services, having been so dismissive, should be dragging their feet now. I made an appointment to see Sandra, my mother's care manager.

I arrived there ready to be magisterial about the whole situation, but Sandra was so pleasant and welcoming that it deflated my imperious facade. A belligerent stance is difficult to maintain in the face of a sunny disposition. The news was good, we could go ahead. I ungraciously wondered how long they'd been sitting on that decision and how long it would have taken Social Services to get in touch with me, had I not made the first move.

I was given the name of a lady who would come and look at the bungalow to see if there were any adaptations needed to the property that Social Services could help with. I was to make an appointment as soon as the bungalow was ours.

We completed on the 9th February, 2001. A letter was sent to the home giving them the statutory four weeks' notice of our intention to take Mum out of there.

13th February, 2001

Re: Mrs Joan C.

Dear Brian,

My brother and I wish to advise you that we are giving four weeks notice of our intention to take Joan out of Huesneath Moor.

As you are probably aware, we have permission from Dr A and Social Services to transfer Joan into my care and we will, all things being well, be fetching her on the afternoon of 16th March 2001.

I would be grateful if all her clothes and other personal effects could be in her room on that day and her medication made available to us.

When Joan came into your care, she brought with her an adjustable table and although she has one in her room, it's not hers. I have no objection to taking that one, but it is of a sturdier (although shabbier) quality than hers and you may prefer to replace her own table back in her room.

We will be cancelling the direct debit arrangement to the home, so the fees for the March period will be paid by cheque direct to Huesneath Moor on receipt of your invoice.

I will be moving home on the 28th February, to provide appropriate accommodation for Joan, so the final invoice will need to be sent to...

Yours sincerely,

I finished work on the 23rd February. I packed up my home, which only amounted to a transit van's worth, and began to gather together all the paraphernalia that would be required for Mum to furnish the bungalow. We had just over two weeks to get everything ready. That should have been a cinch, but it doesn't pay to take anything for granted. I hadn't factored in — the flu.

***

Within forty-eight hours of moving into the bungalow in Water Park Road, I went down with the dreaded lurgy. It wasn't proper flu, I've only had that once in my life, but there is no heroic working through influenza. With a high temperature and every joint in your body on fire, you're in bed and going nowhere. This was just a vicious cold virus. Although I yearned to be in bed, my head was thumping and I felt faint every time I stood upright. I had developed a cough that emanated from someplace deep inside my chest. My ribcage was sore from the effort of moving the cough from its embedded position.

I'd planned to paint Mum's bedroom, but I struggled to stand up, never mind balancing on a ladder wielding a paintbrush and breathing in the fumes. In fairness to the previous owners, the décor was perfectly acceptable, except that all the walls were white, a non-colour, with the sterility of hospital walls. Still, white they had to remain.

While I was noisily dying, consumed with mucus and self pity, the hospital rang to say that they could provide the airwave mattress, but not the bed to put it on. I broke the bad news to Bob. This was an expensive item, but there was no alternative, certainly not at this short notice. We'd have to buy a hospital type bed. I'd already found a firm who supplied them for domestic use. I'd hoped it was a contingency plan we wouldn't have to implement, but at least I didn't have to waste time looking for a supplier.

I made the phone call. Yes, they could supply the bed and they would deliver within three working days. Did I need cot sides? I didn't know. My mother certainly didn't have cot sides at the home, she was using an ordinary bed, which must have been back breaking for staff, as the height couldn't be varied. I was given to understand that Mum couldn't move herself in the bed and had to have her position altered during the night to avoid bedsores.

I declined the offer of cot sides because of the extra cost, plus I had in mind the controversy surrounding the use of them with people who had dementia. There had been cases of patients climbing over the top of raised cot sides, falling and subsequently breaking limbs. This danger wouldn't apply to my mother but it was an ill thought out decision that I'd later regret.

***

The lady from Social Services came round to see if I needed adaptations. I felt I'd got it covered except for a seat for the bath. She decided there wasn't room in the bathroom to fix a seat and get the hoist into the bathroom to make the transfer. I was pretty sure there was a seat in existence that would work, if we removed the side panel of the bath, but I kept quiet.

Liz, one of these overactive, skinny types, was all for constructing a rail, attached to the ceiling that would run from the bedroom to the bathroom, so that Joan could travel in an overhead sling on this monorail from bed to bath. My brain had been working overtime, while she'd been rattling on about this idea that was never going to come to fruition. I'd have to run it past Bob, but I reckoned if we removed the side panel of the bath and if the feet of the hoist would fit underneath, we could transfer Mum from bed to bath in the hoist, and she would remain attached to it while in the bath. I wasn't going to voice this idea to Liz because, technically, the hoist should only be used to transfer from one piece of furniture to another, not for moving people from room to room.

I let Liz depart, with the overhead monorail forefront in her mind. I was fixed on penetrating her grey matter to ensure that I was, at least, going to get the hoist with the slings by the due date. I had the distinct impression that I'd have to reinforce this request with a few reminder phone calls, as she wasn't even able to provide me with a wheelchair until two weeks after Mum was due to arrive.

I wasn't totally convinced about the bath seat not being a viable option, but I thought my idea of using hoist and sling for the whole business was actually preferable. So, of the three items Social Services were supposed to supply, the bath seat had effectively been refused and the wheelchair was unavailable. Only the hoist should actually be in situ when Mum arrived.

***

The first case in Devon of the horrendous 2001 outbreak of foot and mouth disease was announced on the 24th February, 2001. It was heartbreaking, but predictable that the disease would spread. Conspiracy theories were rife throughout Britain and mass cremations were becoming evident as we drove through the countryside to collect Mum. A dark time for our rural communities.

Bob had borrowed a minibus with wheelchair lift at the rear from the residential home where I'd recently worked and had hired a wheelchair for use until the end of the month. Malcolm, a friend of mine, was going to meet us there with his transit van, so we could pick up all Mum's bits of furniture at the same time that we collected her. Once more, Bob called in his mate, Bill, who would assist with the lifting and shifting.

We turned up mob-handed just after lunch. I was still fragile from the aftermath of my cold, but ready or not, this was it. Mum had recovered from her cold and although frail, was alert and deemed fit to travel. The guys stripped the room of all her furniture while she sat in her wheelchair with an intense expression on her face. I explained to her what was happening. How much she understood I'd no idea, but she didn't appear distressed, just transfixed by the activity.

Transit van loaded, I wrapped Mum up in blankets and wheeled her outside with Dr A's warning ringing in my ears.

'You have to understand that Joan is so frail, the move itself might kill her and she may not live more than twenty-four hours.'

It was notable that the only person who spoke to us was the nurse who handed me Mum's medication. By this time relations between management and me had pretty well broken down, there really wasn't anything left to say to each other.

My mother took it all in her stride, I thought she might become anxious and start screaming, but she gave all the indications, as far as she was able to convey emotion, of enjoying the adventure. But then she hadn't been outside for twelve months or more. I really hadn't known what to expect.

Once strapped into the minibus and on our way, she kept reaching out, as if to steady herself, throughout the forty minute journey. I sat next to Mum, constantly reassuring her and talking about her life to come at Water Park Road.

The guys unloaded the transit van and saying he would be back tomorrow, Bob left, with Bill in tow, to return the minibus.

We were on our own, Joan and me. This was it, the start of a new chapter in both our lives and almost certainly the final chapter for my mother.

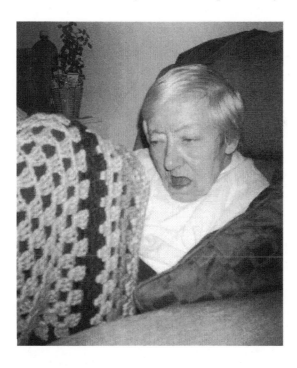

PART 5

Chapter Eighteen

It was a weird feeling. This was my mother, but I didn't really know her, not as she was now. I reverted to care assistant mode. Don't do anything without having explained what you're about to do first and apologise in advance before performing intimate tasks that would be necessary, but not comfortable.

Inevitably, the first few days were stilted. I'd given myself a week with Mum before involving Jodi. I thought in that time I'd be able to develop a routine and a more personal care plan than the generic one that I'd submitted to Dr A. I also knew that we were in the honeymoon period, the behaviour that my mother was exhibiting at the moment would bear no relationship to her conduct in a month's time.

That first week she was very compliant, like a visitor, which was just as well, as this was a learning curve for us both. I was still figuring out the best way to do things. To construct the skeleton of a daily routine, I adhered to my submitted care plan, but revised it as I went along.

Technically, I was supposed to transfer Mum from her recliner in the lounge to the bed, by hoisting her into the wheelchair, take both wheelchair and hoist into the bedroom and then hoist from wheelchair to the bed. This was hard work, time consuming and caused her undue stress. She was rigid and resistant and getting her into a safe position in the wheelchair was difficult and a lot of extra angst for such a short journey to the bedroom. She just wouldn't bend in the middle. I thought this might be anxiety at being handled and may well improve as my mother gained confidence in me.

As the situation stood, I decided to transport her in the hoist sling from recliner to bed. There were a few chunks taken out of the skirting board as I learnt to navigate the hoist through doorways and along the hall. I treated it as a joke every time we collided with the woodwork. By the end of the week, I could do it without hitting anything, or clouting Mum's feet against the door frames.

Another care plan myth was use of the commode. After several attempts, I realised that there was no way she was going to bend at the waist sufficiently to sit, in a constructive position, on the commode and quite honestly I couldn't see the point. She had no control over bladder or bowel, so it'd be down to pot luck and gravity. It wasn't worth the hassle and the obvious distress it was causing her.

I wasn't using the kind of pads that had been in use at the home. I favoured the disposable nappy type, similar to the ones used with babies, except giant sized. They weren't totally leak proof, but they were far more effective than the pads used at the home. My plan, as a rule of thumb, was that Mum should be changed every two hours. With a fluid intake of at least two litres a day, she would need frequent changing, and because it entailed being hoisted onto the bed, her position would be altered regularly. It would help to prevent pressure sores, as would the increase in fluids.

I'd always had a minor obsession about pressure sores. The presence of sores, to me, denoted bad care. Prevention of them is labour intensive, but relatively easy. Once they've developed, they're very difficult to eradicate. I'd worked for a while in a nursing home which was at the pricey end of the market and the local Authority wouldn't fund people to go there.

I'd never, before or since, worked in a place where there were so many spectacular examples of pressure sores. It was distressing and indefensible. The staff, who were keen to improve matters, were demoralised because there were no senior staff taking the lead, therefore continuity of care was nonexistent. In the end, I left. In my letter of resignation to the matron I was very explicit about my reasons for going. That particular matron left soon after I did and returned to the public sector.

***

The use of the hoist and sling worked well in getting Mum in and out of the bath. Bob had removed the side panel and as I'd surmised, the feet of the hoist fitted right underneath the bath, which meant she would hang from the sling, directly over the bath, so I could lower her into the water. Mum remained in the sling, attached to the hoist, all the time she was in the bath. Then I transferred her, covered in towels, back to her bed, over which I'd placed a waterproof sheet with more towels on top. She was dried, then rolled to remove the damp towels and waterproof sheet, then creamed, padded, dressed and hoisted into the lounge.

This was no five minute job, especially when you factored in the suppository insertion and the wait for a result, before the bathing took place. Only once did I misjudge it and Mum took a dump in the bath. That was such a ghastly mistake, I was keen never to risk a repeat performance. After that lesson, I learnt to be more patient and never presumed that there was nothing in the bowel, just because it hadn't happened in the statutory twenty minutes. The increased fluid levels played a part here too, in reducing constipation.

***

We'd reached the end of our first week. Mum had eaten well, but it would take a while to put some padding back onto her emaciated body. I was shocked, seeing her for the first time without clothes on. She looked like a concentration camp survivor, I almost expected to see a tattooed number on her wrist. Every rib could be counted and her shoulder blades were pronounced. I was mortified and angry to see what had happened to her in two years.

It took an hour to feed her, which was three hours a day. There certainly wouldn't be the staff available in that nursing home, or any other that I know of, who would be able to spend that amount of time feeding one resident. Weight loss wasn't a symptom of Alzheimer's disease, as I'd been told. It was the result of malnutrition due to failure to feed the clients in their care. It must still be happening in many care homes today.

Alzheimer's sufferers often have a poor swallow reflex and can choke easily if time isn't taken to prepare food that's easy to swallow and the environment in which they are being fed isn't free of distractions. Baggy clothes, often provided for these clients because of their resistance to having their limbs manipulated, unfortunately hide much of the evidence of malnutrition from the eyes of relatives. The myth that weight loss is part of the disease is expounded, it would seem, as a cover up for neglect. Not the fault of care assistants, many of whom know very little about the specific health problems of the clients in their care, but many care providers have a great deal to answer for.

***

That first week, Mum was put into bed at 5pm where she had her tea, having had her main meal at lunchtime. The hospital bed was a brilliant bit of equipment. It had a hand-held control box which meant I could alter the height, move the back rest to put Mum into a sitting position and even raise her legs if I needed to. At about 7pm, after a face, hands and bum wash and a change of pad, I turned her onto her side in a sleeping position, switched on the side light instead of the main overhead light, put on the radio or a CD, at a low level and left her to it.

I was still experimenting with what worked and what didn't, conscious that this whole episode was going to be a constant re-jigging of procedures as time went on. At the moment this was the plan that Jodi would be working to on her shifts, when I'd be out and she'd be in charge. I left Mum's bedroom door open so she could hear me moving around, clearing up, preparing for tomorrow. Sometimes, she'd chunter to herself, just noises, often with the modulation of speech but no recognisable articulation. When I looked in at 9pm she'd be asleep. I'd turn off the sound and leave her with a night light on.

At about midnight, I'd go in to change her pad and turn her onto her other side. Routinely, she would pass copious amounts or urine before midnight and not a great deal between then and 7am. I started using an absorbent bed pad over the airwave mattress for the first half of the night in an attempt to keep the sheet dry.

The recommendation with this type of mattress is not to put anything over it except a sheet, but the rubberised material of the mattress made Mum sweat, so by midnight she often needed a complete bed change, sheet, nightdress, sometimes duvet cover and always her incontinence pad. I very soon decided that wearing a T-shirt in bed was a more comfortable solution, as her nightdress was often soaked and clinging round her legs. With just a T-shirt, the bed pad drew the urine away from her skin and her T-shirt was short enough to prohibit urine being absorbed by it, except sometimes around the bottom edge and was, in any event, easier to change.

After the midnight ritual, I'd give Mum a drink of water, resettle her, shove the soiled linen into the washing machine in readiness for tomorrow and go to bed. Of course, I was wide awake by this time so often spent the next two hours tossing and turning, unable to switch off. Inevitably, as the weeks went on and I wasn't getting a good night's rest, I'd fall asleep in the recliner during the evening. This actually worked in my favour. I'd be fast asleep in her chair by 10pm. The central heating would go off just after then so the cold would wake me, at around midnight. I'd sort Mum out and then climb into my own bed, not fretting if I didn't sleep immediately, because I'd already banked two hours or more. All psychological, no doubt, but it worked for me.

***

Jodi started her shifts accompanied by Sharnie, her three-year-old daughter. Initially, I had some reservations, but I wanted Jodi to be my mother's carer and was prepared to include Sharnie as part of the package.

Three-year-olds have very few prejudices apart from an instinctive aversion to cooked cabbage. Generally, what's acceptable to mum is acceptable to child. Sharnie accepted Joan unconditionally. That feeling appeared to be mutual. Joan was hugged, spoken to lovingly or chastised with a wag of the finger, depending on the situation at the time and she accepted it all. There was no doubt that Sharnie was an asset and my fears had been totally unfounded.

I'd written up a revised care plan and a daily schedule based on the first week. It wasn't just for Jodi's benefit. I didn't know if, or when, I might have to buy in care for a short or prolonged period. If I had to use an agency, there would be little likelihood of them providing the same carer every time. If I wanted things to be done my way, a care plan kept on display was essential.

I heard no more from Social Services about the monorail. The bath chair idea was never implemented and the commode never utilised, after the first few frustrating attempts. I'd purchased a pressure cushion that was used in Mum's recliner and also in her wheelchair. Social Services provided them, but I wasn't informed of that. I learnt the hard way that if you didn't ask, Social Services wouldn't volunteer information about the availability of equipment.

***

The only meal Mum had in her chair was her main meal at 1pm, both breakfast and tea were given to her in bed. The downside was her startle reflex. This was my terminology, because I was never given an explanation as to why this happened.

Her startle reflex had become acute during the early days of her illness. A plane overhead or a motorbike nearby would startle Joan and make her visibly jump, even though they were heard approaching for some seconds or even minutes before the noise became intrusive. Now, without any recognisable stimuli, her whole body would jerk uncontrollably as if she'd received an electric shock. It was worse in the mornings and looked as if Mum was being jump started with a defibrillator. For the onlooker, it was dramatic, and if she had a mouth full of food or drink, the contents would be projected over an extensive area.

The mornings remained her best time and although this had been pure guesswork in the original care plan, it'd proved true. Routine, intimate procedures were done after breakfast, while her mood remained passive. Dressing and undressing continued to be done on the bed and the morning regimen provided a good opportunity to check for any telltale reddened skin. Her heels and groin were in particular need of constant vigilance.

I was convinced that Mum had an ongoing low grade urinary tract infection, but unless it showed up in a sample, which wasn't easy to acquire, the doctor was reluctant to prescribe antibiotics. That was primarily the reason I insisted on a high fluid intake. At least it diluted her urine and it was certainly noticeable that when she hadn't drunk enough, the result was pee with the consistency of chicken soup and a very repugnant odour.

Getting a pad on was dependent on being able to prise her legs apart far enough to get a pad in between them. Her limbs were fixed and resistant and it would have been impossible to slide a sheet of paper between those thighs. The technique was to bend both legs at the knees, so that her feet were flat on the bed, then putting my hands on the inside of her knees, I would rock Mum from side to side, while gradually pressing her knees apart, until I'd achieved a wide enough gap.

The other region of my mother's body that was particularly vulnerable was her heels, so they were massaged with aqueous cream, morning and evening. Mum only wore socks, except when she was in the wheelchair. But when sitting in her recliner, her feet rested on a genuine sheepskin rug, care of the gift shop at The Big Sheep, which was, as the name implies, a sheep orientated theme park, sited a stone's throw from Water Park Road. I could have purchased a piece of synthetic sheepskin from the chemist but just because it carried a medical label the price was exorbitant and it wasn't nearly as dense.

***

I'd been a frequent visitor to "The Big Sheep" with Jake and friends when he was a youngster. It was home-spun entertainment, not commercialised, but the kids enjoyed the unstructured freedom The Big Sheep offered them. They never tired of visiting, especially at lambing time when there were baby lambs to cuddle and bottle feed.

We'd gained free entry, by default, on one occasion. Jake and I were out walking, exploring public footpaths in the immediate vicinity of home and wandered into a field of young bullocks because the footpath ran through it.

Halfway into the field, the herd of frisky and curious bullocks stampeded towards us from the rear. We hared across the rough pasture, running for our lives. The only obvious route was towards the far edge of the field, so we raced towards it, with me praying that there was going to be a way out. The field ended in a steep bank down into a stream. With the cows still in pursuit, we slid down the bank into the water.

Jake was exhilarated by the whole experience. I stood petrified, heart in mouth, unsure what to do next, convinced we'd narrowly escaped death. The herd stopped at the top, staring down at us, their eyes full of menace. One intrepid bullock decided to chance his hoof and came after us down the bank. We both scrambled up the opposite side and forged a gap through a hedge. Breathless and soaked with sludgy water, we found ourselves in the grounds of The Big Sheep. Jake wanted to stay and play, I wanted to go home. I won.

Chapter Nineteen

My mother had an appreciative appetite and in only a few weeks had noticeably gained weight. It was during the lengthy feeding stints that I realised she was more intellectually responsive than I'd first thought. I have to admit that when it was just the two of us, I would invariably carry on a running commentary, not expecting a response, just thinking out loud and talking to myself, which I still do, only now my dog has to listen to it all.

Mum's swallow reflex was slow and she'd choke easily over certain things. Hot beverages were the worst, she usually recovered herself without intervention, but it looked and sounded critical. Possibly, because she feared choking, Mum could be adamantly opposed to drinking anything, and developed the knack of sticking her tongue into the spout of the lid of her drinking cup.

I was willing to respect her right to refuse food, but her intake of fluids was non-negotiable. So I'd have to insert my finger into her mouth, thankful that she had no teeth, gently pull her cheek out and insert the spout into the side of her mouth and into the inside of her cheek. She seemed not to be so prone to choking this way. Hot drinks were still a challenge, but Mum had always loved her cup of tea and I didn't want to deprive her of that pleasure just yet.

I had to start the feeding process with the request, 'Open,' or 'Big mouth'.

Much as you would with a young child, I was certain that she understood the phrase because she wouldn't open her mouth, although I was hovering with the spoon near her lips, until I issued the command. When she'd had enough, Mum would clamp her mouth shut. If I asked, 'Enough?' or 'Finished?' sometimes she would very quietly say, 'Yes' or 'Umm' or just nod her head once. Blink and you'd miss it but I was always delighted if I got a response. Similarly, if she was just resting in between mouthfuls, but wanted more, she would sometimes say, 'No' or shake her head very slightly. But there were no guarantees that there would be any response at all.

To cater for my mother's dietary needs meant I had to cook, a skill that I'd let slide since leaving the marital home. I'd never been a foodie, its essential fuel but I can't get excited about it. Now I had to try to put myself in my mother's skin. What was going to appeal to her palate when presented in a liquidised form?

Inevitably, my freezer became full of portions of the basic elements of meals. Liquidised chicken, beef, pork and fish ready to convert into a gourmet meal by the addition of a frozen sauce and frozen liquidised vegetables, except potatoes, which were freshly cooked. I'd have a cooking evening, devoted to producing mushy food to feed the freezer which was beginning to take on the appearance of a science laboratory's specimen storage facility. I bought sweet stuff, mainly yoghurts, mousse, custard, mini trifles and cakes or sponges in tins.

My own meals were provided on a much more ad hoc basis. Nutritionally speaking, I didn't eat as well as I should have done, it was too easy to just slump at the end of the day, with a ready meal, coffee and whatever sweet stuff took my fancy.

Jodi and I developed an easy and successful working partnership. As an added bonus Jodi was a trained hairdresser and was happy to cut Mum's hair, which was another potential problem resolved. Taking my mother to a hairdresser wasn't a realistic option. I'd been prepared to cut it myself, after all I did my own. But my hairdressing skills extended to one style, a crop, which varied in length according to how depressed I felt at the time. Depression, strangely enough, always gave me the urge to cut my hair. I'd toyed with the idea of a mobile hairdresser coming to the bungalow, but if my mother wasn't in an amenable mood, it would have taken a special stylist to stay the course.

***

Six months after I'd moved in with my mother, I sold her little red Ford Fiesta to Jeremy, her former hairdresser. He came round to the bungalow to pay and collect the car. The deal was done in the living room where Mum was seated in her recliner, chattering quietly to herself. Jeremy's discomfort was palpable. He was unable to even acknowledge her existence in the room.

I should have felt sorry for him, but I didn't, because by then I'd realised that quite a lot of people I'd thought of as friends were uncomfortable around Mum and didn't know how to react. They'd visit once, but never again. I often felt isolated, but it was my mother's home and I wasn't prepared to shove her in the bedroom every time we had a visitor. Six months on and that was no longer an issue. Apart from Jake and Bob, we didn't have visitors and it was a situation I naively hadn't foreseen.

***

By the end of April, spring had decided to begin and so had my mother's "inappropriate vocalisation". The honeymoon period was coming to an end. Noise levels were increasing, so much so I became concerned that the neighbours would think I was beating Joan to a pulp and call the police. It didn't help that the elderly man who lived next door was an ex-policeman.

Bill lived by himself, but was often visited by a young police constable who lived at the top of the road. Bill was as deaf as a post, but his friend, the police constable wasn't, and every time his car pulled up outside, I was in anxious expectation of the knock at the door.

I asked my neighbours on the other side if they could hear the shouting. Roy and Eileen were ideal neighbours, I couldn't have asked for better. Eileen was a physiotherapist with the re-ablement team and Roy was simply a genuinely gentle guy with prostate problems. Yes, they could hear her shouting, but they were quick to reassure me.

'It's not a problem, honestly,' Roy said.

I scrutinised the drugs Mum was taking. Mrs B's 'no unnecessary drugs' stand had obviously been blown out of the water when Brian took over. She was on a daily cocktail of Paroxetine, Mellaril, Lorazepam and Lactulose for her bowels. I hadn't changed any of these because, up to now, the shouting problem hadn't really been an issue, but I didn't know if these particular drugs were appropriate or not. I wasn't told why they'd been prescribed, and I certainly had no clear idea why my mother was shouting. Jodi and I brainstormed the problem but didn't come up with anything conclusive. We thought it was maybe due to:

Discomfort: A difficult one. Joan could have been experiencing muscle cramps or spasms, stomach pains, constipation, UTI or just an itch that needed scratching. We didn't know and she couldn't tell us.

Boredom: A very possible contender. We worked at enhancing her living space with use of music, radio, Sharnie's antics, massage and physiotherapy, but with her sight, intellect and movement severely compromised there were limitations. Now the weather was warmer, we decided that short trips out in the wheelchair might help, if boredom was the culprit.

Frustration: With all her problems, I'd have been surprised if she wasn't frustrated. Neither of us had much of a clue how much intellect or awareness there was left intact. Personally, I hoped that there was very little, the thought of a high level of awareness trapped within a non-responsive body was unbearable to contemplate. We always tried to talk to Joan as if she was able to comprehend everything and had an opinion.

Habit: Joan had been allowed to scream herself into a state of exhaustion at Huesneath Moor and they simply shut her away in her room when it got too much. But then why had she been relatively quiet for the first two months here?

I decided a visit to the doctor might be expedient, because I couldn't see myself being able to tolerate the shouting and screaming if the levels increased much more. The doctor was concerned and sympathetic. He raised his eyebrows, but made no adverse comment as he referred to his computer screen and scrutinised the medication Joan was taking. He suggested that the drugs could be making the shouting problem worse, as they sometimes aggravated the symptoms they were prescribed to alleviate. He wanted me to take Joan off the Mellaril. For some reason that he didn't elaborate on, he wasn't happy about prescribing it for Joan. It would have to be done gradually, but he thought it might improve matters and didn't feel that there was any merit in her continuing to take it.

I was prepared to try his suggestion, with reservations. After all, Mum had probably been put on this drug because of the shouting and screaming. It might not make her condition worse by taking her off Mellaril, but I had little confidence that it would improve the situation.

***

122

There were three issues that required attention. Namely, sort out someone to take over the Sunday duty from Jodi, find a respite care provider, and make a start on converting an overgrown allotment into a garden worthy of the Chelsea Flower Show. The first two required talking to people, so I made a start on the garden space.

I'd already drawn out a plan, so on paper I had a garden. Now, all I could see ahead was hard work but as the daylight hours became longer I was glad to get out there. It was an escape from the increase in my mother's vocal athletics.

The plan was to split the garden into sections and take each plot as a separate project, otherwise it would have been overwhelming. On good days, I would wrap her up in warm clothes and wheel her outside for a while, to supervise the work. As far as it was possible to tell, she appeared to enjoy it. At least she stopped shouting. Missy, the cat, decided that Mum's lap was a warm seat and made a beeline for her every time she emerged from the lean-to greenhouse, like royalty coming to inspect the loyal serf at work.

Slowly, a garden began to evolve, I had the aches, pains and scratches to prove it. The brambles had been pulled up and a portion of field left to replicate a lawn. Well, it was green, and if I kept it cut short and it wasn't inspected too closely, it would pass as a lawn. Around the edges I created irregular areas of interest with judicious use of planting, gravel, paving slabs, sand and some mammoth rocks selected at the local quarry and hauled into place, piece by piece, to create a rockery. Viewing Alan Titchmarsh on the TV hadn't been in vain. The only discernible difference was that he had staff, a healthy budget and charisma.

I did leave one legacy of its former existence as an allotment, a row of espalier conference pear trees along one fence and tayberries along another. It looked very easy on paper, but the project took the best part of six months to complete.

***

The garden was an endeavour that I had under control, finding respite care for my mother was not. I was beginning to despair of finding anywhere. Nursing homes in the area didn't have designated respite beds. Why would they? The idea was to fill all the beds, all the time.

I compiled a list of every nursing home I could find within a reasonable distance. A couple of homes were happy to take Mum for a week's respite care if they happened to have an empty bed, but I wanted to book in advance so that I could have a week's break every three months and I wanted my first break in June. Only one home could match my requirements and assured me that I could book ahead, they would make a bed available and the shouting wouldn't be a problem. So, with a choice of only one, I booked a bed for June.

This nursing home was one I'd contemplated moving my mother into before I'd made the decision to care for her myself. The matron hadn't returned my call, as had been promised, so I'd discounted it. Time would tell if I'd made the right decision. The next problem was how to transport Mum from home to home.

I'd been toying with the idea of purchasing a suitable vehicle for a while. I was now taking my mother, in her wheelchair, on regular afternoon jaunts around the housing estate. Londonderry Estate had expanded over the years and was still growing, so there were plenty of streets and connecting footpaths to walk, but not the most scintillating scenery.

My mother had confounded Dr A's prognosis and was becoming stronger and was continuing to gain weight. As she did so, she appeared to take more notice of her surroundings and seemed to enjoy her outings. The question was, how could I extend this positive experience? The obvious answer was a vehicle that took a wheelchair with its user in situ, to allow us to travel further afield. I broached the subject with Bob, who promised to give it some thought.

He got back to me a couple of days later with a possible solution. His mate Bill, the same guy who'd helped with the moves, had left his job as a bus driver and was now working in a garage that also sold secondhand cars and vans. The garage had a relatively elderly Skoda van, which had been taking up space for a while, and they were willing to sell it at a reasonable price.

While Jodi was on duty, I went with Bob to take a look. This style of van had a separate cab which meant you couldn't access the body of the van from the cab, only from the rear doors. That allowed for increased headroom, high enough to accommodate someone sitting in a wheelchair. There was a window that allowed the driver to see behind, into the van, sliding windows on the sides and windows in the rear doors. Potentially, a veritable popemobile.

Better yet, the guys at the garage said they knew where to buy a kit that would provide anchor points in the back, a special seatbelt and ramps and they were able to fit it. In addition, they would remove the connecting window to allow me to talk to Mum and also permit heat, from the cab, to filter backwards. They'd done this cheap conversion before. Two weeks later, my mother was the owner of a converted Skoda Van. It was a poor man's lash-up, but it worked.

***

Jodi was covering as many of the Sunday shifts as she could, but I knew her partner wanted her at home at the weekends. I needed to find a carer who could cover the shifts allowing me to continue to attend the Sunday meeting at the Kingdom Hall. Meeting attendance had been the backbone of my life for a long time now, and I really needed to keep the spiritual aspects of my life in place.

I put an advert in the local paper and had two phone calls in response. The first girl who rang claimed to have experience looking after the elderly. I asked her where she'd worked and was given the name of the home that Mum had recently vacated. Then it clicked, her name and Huesneath Moor in the same frame. She was a young lass, only about seventeen or eighteen. She'd been accused of theft and was dismissed from the home. It was petty stuff, clothes and toiletries, taken from the residents. For reasons best known to those involved, the police were never informed, she was simply asked to leave. Mum may have been one of her victims, brand new M&S T-shirts had gone missing, even though her name tag was sewn into them. From experience, I knew that name tags didn't prevent clothes from disappearing. My mother had been the recipient of all sorts of odd garments, some obviously meant for men. I would root them out of her room on a regular basis. That's why I hadn't attached any suspicion to the disappearance of the newly acquired T-shirts.

Needless to say, I terminated the conversation in the most diplomatic way possible. I was, in any event, looking for somebody of more mature years who had experience in the care of people with advanced dementia. I felt an element of sympathy for her. Although not the sharpest knife in the drawer, she'd been a pleasant girl, as far as I recalled, but she'd be here on her own. It was a risk I wasn't willing to take.

The only other applicant for this prestigious position was a more mature woman, in age anyway, and I knew her. I'd worked with her several times in different homes. Care work is like that. If you work in that field for long enough, your path will inevitably cross with the same people, in different places. Tessa was something of a rough diamond, but a competent carer, whose heart was in the right place.

Tessa took over the Sunday duties which simply extended her weekend sleep-in night duty at a nearby residential home. She got paid more for the three hours with Mum than for an entire night at the care home. I was appalled when she told me what the hourly rate was. True, she was allowed to sleep, but you're always on red alert and some nights it could be pretty frantic with never a wink of sleep to be had. I wondered if it was legal to pay such low wages for a ten-hour shift, now that the National Minimum Wage was in operation.

***

Now we were mobile, we were out somewhere most days. The technique required for getting Mum into the van was learnt by trial and error, bearing in mind it all took place in the street in full view of the curtain twitchers, a club of which I was now a fully paid-up member. Any disturbance, a voice, barking dog and I was there, inspecting the street, searching for a distraction to my routine existence.

I put on a show for Water Park Road, though not by choice. The ramps had to be placed at the correct distance apart, then I had to line up Mum and wheelchair with the ramps. From then on it was a leap of faith as I took a run at it to gain just enough momentum to push her up the ramps and into the van, too much propulsion and she'd be up the ramps and into the driver's seat. At the start, I often failed to make the gradient on the first attempt, but slowly I became more proficient at it and quite blasé about the whole performance.

We didn't go far, I was aware that it was probably a fairly bumpy ride in the back of the van. We had our regular haunts. Victoria Park, Westward Ho!, Appledore Quay and Bideford Town were all utilised to the full. It was no coincidence that they all had Hockings Ice Cream vans in operation. I'd take a spoon and copious tissues and spoon-feed my mother with their delicious ice cream.

***

I'd like to announce that Joan ceased to scream while we were out and about. Sadly, that wasn't the case, though I was uncertain if it was entirely unrelated to events. I recall a walk along the promenade at Westward Ho! We were stuck behind a large family, who meandered along the promenade, devouring chips. They filled the entire width of the walkway, oblivious to other pedestrians' attempts to pass in either direction. I'd spent a few minutes behind this impenetrable mass of flesh as I tried in vain to find a gap. Joan, by accident or design, let out an ear splitting scream. The family parted like the biblical Red Sea and with a smile and a cheery 'thank you' we sailed through, my mother's screams, caught on the wind, ebbed and flowed behind us.

On another occasion I had this crazy idea of going to Rosemoor, a very attractive RHS garden with different themed areas, and as this was in June, a beautiful rose garden in full bloom, a delight to the senses. Rosemoor is in Torrington, with hindsight just a little too far to travel in the back of a van along a road noted for its bends.

Possibly, the journey had been too arduous, though we'd been to Torrington town before without incident, but Rosemoor was a smidge further out. Joan was quiet, until I'd parted with the entrance fee. As soon as we got into the gardens, she started. My mother shouted and screamed without a pause to draw breath. I wheeled her, sat on a bench with her and took her to the rose garden to inhale the perfume. Nothing was working in my favour. After less than an hour, out of embarrassment, frustration and concern that there might actually be something seriously amiss, we left. As soon as Joan was back in the van, she stopped. We never tried the Rosemoor experience again.

Her very favourite place was Atlantic Village, a factory outlet retail park, a stone's throw from home. She was happy to be wheeled around the shops. Mum would put out her hand to touch the clothes in the Edinburgh Woollen Mill shop and chunter softly to herself or possibly me, who knows? I'd answer, as if her unintelligible chatter was directed at me, but never noticed a response that indicated she meant it to be interactive.

Atlantic Village was a useful and convenient all-weather destination. It was used often for the days when I was going stir crazy, or the screaming was penetrating the ear plugs I'd taken to using, to protect myself from this auditory assault.

***

I was able to provide Jodi with a minimum of fifteen hours work a week. Most weeks it was more, averaging out to about eighteen hours. Jodi had kept her two nights at the residential home and these extra hours boosted her income equivalent to at least another one and a half nights. She seemed happy with the arrangement.

Jodi was now busy arranging her wedding for September and wanted Mum to be there. I was touched by this totally impractical gesture. I pointed out that the bride was supposed to be the focal point of the day, not the screaming banshee in the wheelchair. When she was screaming at full force, Joan must have exceeded eighty-five on the decibel scale. Jodi and I came to an agreement that, if it was possible, I'd be outside the registry office with Mum, when Jodi emerged as a married woman.

Jodi was genuinely fond of my mother, which was an unexpected bonus. As a carer, it isn't an automatic response to like all the clients who you're paid to look after. Hopefully, you're able to hide your feelings and still give care that's competent and compassionate. You'll always have your favourites and it never ceases to amaze me that it's not one type fits all. The guy I might find totally obnoxious will be someone else's favourite, the little old lady who aims a kick or a clout at you every time you come within striking distance might appeal to me, but others would give her a wide berth. As the screaming showed little signs of abating, I had begun to find my own mother pretty obnoxious and wanted to give her an extremely wide berth, preferably in a sound-proofed room.

Chapter Twenty

My first week's respite was mid-June and I was more than ready for the break. I drove Mum there without incident, although the home was further away than I'd have liked. I settled her into her bedroom, sorted her cassette/radio out, put away her clothes and toiletries and sat with Mum until somebody came. Only they didn't. My mother had been sitting in her wheelchair for long enough. She needed to be transferred to her bed and probably required changing. I waited for the best part of an hour, then went in search of someone, anyone. I found the nurse in charge of that floor and explained the situation, of which she knew nothing. Flustered and furrowed of brow, she disappeared to vent her spleen on some unsuspecting administrator.

An hour later, I was ready to leave. I had misgivings about leaving Mum there as, so far, I'd been less than impressed. On the way out I was waylaid by the matron. She wanted a word with me before I left. Hoping she hadn't the ability to read minds, because mine was disgruntled and focused on escape, I dutifully followed her to the office.

Basically, she just wanted to complete the paperwork. Was there any food that Joan disliked? Any allergies? What was her daily routine? I kept a straight face knowing that whatever routine Joan was used to would not be considered. She'd be shoe-horned into the existing regime of the home. The matron briefly met my glazed gaze.

'We operate a policy of non-resuscitation, unless otherwise instructed. How do you feel about that?'

I hadn't seen that one coming. I wasn't sure if that was the standard policy in nursing homes generally. I'd worked in them, Joan had been a resident in one, but I didn't recall ever having this discussion before. I agreed to the policy, signed on the dotted line and left.

＊＊

During my week's respite I went to see the doctor. I really needed some help. I was finding the shouting and especially the screaming, difficult to tolerate. I could feel myself sinking back into the depressive state I'd experienced when looking after my mother the first time around.

Having been off antidepressants for two years, I felt depressed at the thought of being depressed. To me it signalled failure. My blood pressure was up again, so inevitably he recommended that I go back on antidepressants and promised that he'd refer Joan to a psychologist who specialised in the care of the elderly.

I waited for him to tell me that I was an idiot for putting myself in this situation in the first place, but he didn't. He told me that I was doing an incredible job and how much he admired me for taking it on. I'd like to say that I blossomed at these kind remarks, but I simply burst into tears, fuelled by exhaustion and guilt. I didn't feel that I was doing a good job at all. Trish had been right, I couldn't cope, whatever had made me think that I could? I felt as if I'd failed Mum and myself all over again.

***

I collected my mother on the following Wednesday. Her eyes were virtually glued shut and she looked awful. Her face was blotchy and sore, where the staff had likely used soap, although her notes were explicit in their request that soap shouldn't be used. Once we were home and I'd undressed her, I wasn't impressed by her obvious weight loss and evidence of urine burn. I found it hard to comprehend how she'd ended up in this state in the space of a week. I really didn't know if I could put her through it again. The travel and the experience had taken its toll.

By Friday, bad care or not, I was almost on the verge of sending her back. She'd slept virtually all day, now at 1.15am she was shouting at the top of her voice. I'd been in and changed her, watered her and altered her position, but I suppose Mum had already banked her quota of sleep. I wished I could say the same.

***

The next day we had a surprise visit from the Birmingham contingency. My mother's two sisters and a niece turned up at the bungalow. They were on holiday at Hartland for a week. Mum, having been awake most of the night, was in a subdued mood and showed no glimmer of recognition. The visit happened around her rather than involving her.

They left with the promise that they'd ring me the next day and arrange to meet up for lunch, perhaps at Appledore. My heart sank. While the idea of lunch out with my mother sounded plausible to the uninitiated, the logistics were not. All that loomed before me was a massive headache.

Having spent the following morning on tenterhooks, awaiting the telephone call, the Birmingham clan didn't contact me until well after Mum had eaten her lunch, so I arranged to meet them for afternoon tea. It was an idyllic summer's day, with sun that warmed and comforted, without the humid heat that so often makes summer days so draining. We sat at one of the tables set up on the street, outside a tea shop on the quay. I waited with Mum, while Olive and Barbara purchased tea and cakes.

An elderly gentleman with Nordic poles and a substantial rucksack sat himself down with a cappuccino at the next table. He volunteered the information that he was walking from Land's End to John O'Groats. The man was obviously post-retirement and admitted that he was using his bus pass to traverse places of little interest and had stayed some nights in guest houses and pubs rather than his tent. He had, he said, all the time in the world to take the opportunity to enjoy the country that he'd lived in all his life, but knew so little about. Discreet enquiry, on my part, revealed that he was seventy-three, older than I'd thought.

It occurred to me that the old lady seated by my side, her fingers playing in the air, totally immersed in her own universe, the lady who I once knew as my mother, had been well along the Alzheimer's route at seventy-three. What, I contemplated, would she have achieved, in the intervening years since my father's death, if she hadn't fallen foul of this disease? How would life pan out for this eloquent gentleman who sat, head back, eyes closed, absorbing the sun's rays? Was it totally indiscriminate, by the roll of the dice, who developed Alzheimer's and who didn't?

It wasn't until some years later when talking to Olive, I learnt that her father, my grandfather, who'd died with a heart attack before I was born, had already become senile, although only in his early sixties. Coincidence or genetics? There is now evidence that early onset dementia of the Alzheimer's type, which develops before the age of sixty-five, is often genetic and that the faulty gene can be passed on. A deadly inheritance.

That night, after Mum was safely tucked up in bed, I made a mug of coffee and took it into the back garden. Sitting with my back against her bedroom wall and with Dire Straits in my headset, I let the tears flow into the warm dusk until the stars came out.

***

I went out for a meal with my aunts and cousin on the last evening of their holiday. It was my regular three hours off-duty which I used to attend my meeting, so Jodi was coming in anyway. Unfortunately, it was my choice of venue, based on a recommendation, not personal experience. The food, apart from my cousin's meal, left a lot to be desired. Judging by the lack of customers in what I knew to be a popular restaurant, I think it must have been the chef's night off.

Olive was openly disgruntled about it and I thought at one point that things were going to turn nasty. Admittedly, the food was rubbish, but if you're not prepared to complain to the right people, you might as well make the most of it. Olive was still venting her dissatisfaction about it the next morning, when they popped in to say goodbye on their way home. As if I didn't feel bad enough.

That evening, Mum was very restless, still moaning and chuntering at 11.30pm. By 12.30am the low level noise had escalated to screams. I could tolerate her vocal solo during the day, but since her week in respite care she'd had disturbed nights almost every night, and if Joan was awake, then so was I.

When I went into my mother to change and re-position her, she was wide awake and continued to shout. Having done all I could do and feeling that there wasn't anything wrong, I decided to turn off her night-light in the hope that the darkened room would help her to sleep. I toyed with the idea of giving her a sleeping tablet, but it would still be a couple of hours before it kicked in and then Joan would be zapped until lunchtime. A vicious circle.

By the time I was ready for bed, Joan was still yelling and my stomach was in a knot. I'd given her paracetamol, now I was afraid to go back into her room. Afraid because the way I felt at that moment, I could easily have hurt her. I understood how a mother could be driven into shaking her baby to death. No, I couldn't go back in there, not tonight.

When I went into her room the next morning, my mother was on the floor. Major guilt trip. She'd stopped shouting at about 1.30am and I didn't go back into her room then in case I woke her up! I'd no idea how long she'd been on the floor. By her position, Mum had toppled forward. She had marks on her knees and her head was at the bottom end of the bed as she lay on the carpet. There didn't appear to be anything broken but she was icy cold. I hoisted her back onto the bed and attempted to warm her up.

It was amazing really, three months ago Mum wasn't able to move at all in bed and I never dreamt I would need cot sides. This was supposed to be a deteriorating condition. It highlighted that her weakness had been entirely due to enforced immobility and malnutrition. None of this alleviated my sense of guilt one bit. I should have checked her after she quietened down.

I rang the local Health Authority to see if they could provide cot sides for the bed. They didn't have them in store and, in any event, they didn't provide them for dementia cases. I knew that, but she was never going to be able to climb over the top of cot sides, but I had the feeling that falling out of bed would become an established pattern if I didn't do something to prevent it. I rang the firm who sold us the bed, but a machine kicked in to announce that they finished work at lunchtime on Friday and I'd have to ring back on Monday.

I finally got Joan warmed up by bedtime. I had to sponge her feet with warm water to bring them back to life, but she seemed none the worse for her hypothermic experience and remarkably there wasn't a bruise on her. On the plus side, she was quiet throughout the day and slept through the night. Once she was in bed, I dragged the mattress from the spare bed into her room and put it on the floor next to her, in case there was a repeat performance.

The following night, Joan yelled on and off virtually all night. When I went into her room for the umpteenth time at 3.15am, she'd swung her legs out of the bed again and was on her way to the floor. It was as if she'd learnt a new skill and now she was going to keep practising until she got it right. Before Joan had her week's respite care she was sleeping through the night, since returning home she'd become an insomniac. I'd noticed that her sleep had been getting lighter, she'd become easier to disturb. I'd surmised that reducing the Mellaril, as the doctor had requested, probably accounted for that, but what was the answer? We couldn't go on like this. The birds outside were in full voice before I got to sleep that night.

The cot sides were delivered and installed, so further attempts to spend her nights on the floor were thwarted, but the shouting and screaming continued to increase. Now it was becoming a regular night problem, as well as throughout the day.

I felt that it was possibly a UTI. The doctor gave me a short course of antibiotics and Mum did quieten down, but he refused to prescribe again when the urine sample came back clear. That was understandable, although my instinct was that she might have a permanent low grade infection and I seriously wondered if she needed to be on antibiotics permanently. When Mum had the frequent short courses of them, it always improved her mood, but that didn't appear to be an acceptable form of long-term treatment. The only thing I could do was keep her fluids up to the two litres a day mark, or more.

Although there were no more nightly excursions, Mum continued to scream and shout throughout the day and night, taking time out for meals. I received a letter from the psychologist. In it he said:

I understand that unfortunately your mother has dementia and has periods when she becomes quite agitated and cries out. Your GP has asked if I will be able to discuss this with you to see if there is anything we can do to help.

He wanted to do a home visit on the 20th July. I was a tad sceptical, but desperate. I only hoped that Mum would provide a true picture and not clam up. I needn't have worried.

The night before the visit, I had to give her a sleeping tablet, which I'd wanted to avoid as I didn't want her in a drug-induced stupor for the psychologist's visit. I felt I hadn't got much choice. She was screaming to the point where I could hear the strain on her throat and her voice would almost disappear into a croak. But she kept on, until all her breath had gone and her face has turned purple. Then the screaming would turn into a coughing fit, she would recover and the whole cycle would begin again. Why?

Something had to give. I'd begun to exhibit the stress symptoms which had been the prelude to me cracking up before. I was angry at everyone, had constant digestive problems, acid reflux and a face full of acne that any sixteen-year-old would sympathise with. Pure and simple stress overload.

The psychologist arrived at 11.30am and Joan was already tuned up to top volume. He acknowledged that he could hear her as he got out of his car. She kept it up for the entire proceedings and only calmed down to eat lunch. The psychologist, a pleasant and disarmingly boyish guy, came up with potential reasons why Joan was screaming her way through life. Most of the theories he expounded Jodi and I had already discussed but it was nice to have it confirmed by the expert.

We were expected to explore all these theoretical avenues and as a last resort, drug her. Whether my sanity could withstand this voyage of discovery was open to question. The full recommendations would follow in about two weeks. Whether I could last two more weeks was also questionable. The stress had shortened my fuse by yards.

Towards the end of July, while shopping in Morrison's supermarket, I ran into Louise, my ally at HM. She told me that the home had now changed its use to a business totally unrelated to the care of the elderly. So the decision to move Mum out of that home would have come anyway not long after we'd moved her. Whether we'd made a wise decision, I wasn't in the right frame of mind to contemplate and fortunately Louise didn't ask.

Chapter Twenty-One

By the end of July, I'd received a copy of the letter that the clinical psychologist had sent the GP:

Thank you for your referral of this lady with dementia, whose episodes of shouting are causing considerable distress to her daughter. Mrs C has been living at home with her daughter since 17th March. Previous to this she was in a local nursing home but her daughter removed her from this as she was so unhappy with the care being provided. I understand that the registration officer has in fact upheld four out of five complaints against the home in relation to Mrs C's care.

Presentation

When I arrived, Mrs C was reclined in a chair. She appeared to be aware of my presence and made clear eye contact. However, vocalisations began almost immediately. These largely took the form of extremely loud screaming, whilst leaning forwards with her tongue protruding. She became very flushed in the face and the shouting appeared to purvey emotions of anger/frustration. Mrs C's daughter clearly finds this very upsetting and, indeed, I also found it very aversive. The vocalisations usually start at about 10am and can continue throughout the entire day. They do not appear to occur in conjunction with any particular activity and are usually entirely absent during meal times and personal care. The shouting appears to have got significantly worse over the last month, reaching a point where Mrs C's daughter is finding it very difficult to cope.

General Issues

Mrs C appears to eat well and her sleep pattern appears normal. The only change is that it now takes until about 9pm to settle her whilst originally she would have been asleep by 7pm. Her appetite is good and she has gained weight since leaving the nursing home. Initially, upon returning home from the nursing home, her vocalisations were fairly minimal. However, in more recent weeks they have escalated more dramatically. Mrs C has had long term problems with her bowels and I understand that she has a suppository about every three days. The vocalisations appear to have started since the beginning of her being given a suppository but this may not be particularly significant. She does not show any distress whilst the suppository is being administered and the medication does appear to be very effective in keeping her bowels regular. One would expect, therefore, that the suppository would be helping to reduce rather than increase any vocalisations. Mrs C doesn't engage in any activity during the day and her daughter is finding it increasingly difficult to interact with her. Mrs C did appear to be quite alert to her environment for example following her daughter with her eyes when she moved around the room or went into the kitchen.

Possible Causes

In my experience there are a number of possible causes of this sort of behaviour.

1. UTI.

I understand that Mrs C is currently being tested for a UTI with her daughter reporting that her mother's urine is often very strong and has an offensive smell. Certainly this is quite a common cause of problematic vocalisations and I will be interested to hear whether in fact infection is present.

2. Pain/Discomfort.

The aversive nature of Mrs C's vocalisations is suggestive of distress. However, if she was in marked discomfort one would have expected her appetite to be poor and for the vocalisations not to cease during mealtimes and at night.

3. Medication.

I note from your letter that this lady is prescribed Melleril, Lorazepam and Paroxetine. At present, these do not seem to be effective in controlling her symptoms. I also wonder whether the medication might not in itself be contributing to the problem. Although sedative medication can be effective in controlling such vocalisations, it can also, paradoxically, sometimes result in an increase in such problems. I have come across cases where the medication appears to have increased rather than reduced agitation. Should the medication continue to prove ineffective I think there may well be scope to reduce the Melleril further just to see if this helps. I also wonder whether we might consider if she still needs the Seroxat (Paroxetine).

4. Recent History.

It is clear that Mrs C's daughter feels that she received very poor care indeed in her nursing home. She told me that her mother was left soaked in urine and that she was often excluded from other patients. A general response to this lady's vocalisations appears to have been to isolate her. Also the vocalisations were disturbing to other residents who clearly indicated their anger at Mrs C. I think, therefore, it is fair to say that over the last few years she has been in a significantly aversive environment which would have been likely to increase the distressing vocalisations. It would not be uncommon for such vocalisations to temporarily disappear once the person was moved to a more comfortable environment. However, such vocalisations often re-occur once the person has settled in a new environment. I think, therefore, that we should bear in mind that what we are dealing with may be the result of prolonged poor care and under-stimulation. In this sense it may have become quite an established pattern in her life and one that may be very difficult to reduce.

5. Stimulation

Under-stimulation is often implicated in these sorts of cases. Mrs C's daughter is doing a remarkable job in coping with her mother but clearly cannot provide a particularly stimulating environment. This sort of under-stimulation often leads to repetitive, stereotype behaviours such as problematic vocalisations.

I have said to Mrs C's daughter that we need to adopt a team approach to tackling this problem i.e. Mrs S, yourself and myself. She is well aware that it may take some time for us to be able to make any difference to these vocalisations but understands that there are a wide range of factors that may be contributing to the problem. However, if the vocalisations continue at the same intensity, I think the daughter will need additional support. Obviously our first port of call would be the hypothesis with regard to a UTI or evidence of other infection. It very much sounds as if she does have an infection on a fairly chronic basis. Secondly, I think it would be well worth reviewing her medication with a view to a reduction rather than increase. I would certainly favour reviewing both the Melleril and the Seroxat. I think my third hypothesis would be in relation to the care that this lady has received over the last three years, leading to under-stimulation and possible stereotypic vocalisations. This would mean looking at how we can improve the level of stimulation to this lady without putting further stress on her daughter. It was certainly noticeable that when Mrs C's attention was engaged in something, the vocalisations largely ceased. Depression and undiagnosed pain seem to me less likely explanations but can still be borne in mind.

I think Mrs S is well aware there is unlikely to be a straight forward solution to this problem. In fact, I think that we may have to intervene on a number of levels to produce any significant change. Our initial plan of action, therefore, would be to treat any infection, review her medication and begin to explore ways of providing her with a more stimulating and engaging environment.

I would very much welcome a chance to talk this case over with you and will be in contact by phone within the next few days to see if we can arrange a meeting at a convenient time.

***

I handed the letter over to Jodi without comment. She read it through with a reaction that veered from nods of agreement to snorts of derision.

'Did he actually suggest what more we could possibly do to provide this stimulating environment?'

I shook my head slowly, denoting despair and disbelief. We were doing as much as we could. Joan's posture was fixed and rigid and she disliked being manhandled. We played music, Sharnie was very interactive with Joan and would step in where angels feared to tread and give her a resounding telling off when the shouting moved up a gear. She was taken out every day, weather permitting, and would still shout. We gave her a massage and physiotherapy, to try to reduce the rigidity in her limbs, but she shouted through that and all other aspects of her personal care, except having food put in her mouth. What else could we do? We needed constructive advice as to other activities we could employ, but that wasn't forthcoming.

By the time I'd received the letter, I'd already been refused antibiotics for a UTI because nothing showed up in a laboratory test. I agreed that it probably was a chronic infection, but if the GP wouldn't prescribe, it was stalemate.

Parts of the summary of our discussion at the time were inaccurate. Mum was never expected to be asleep before 9pm, but was now having increasingly noisy and broken nights and the only action that had stopped the shouting, while the psychologist was present, was feeding her with lunch.

I'd already reduced the Melleril which had simply made matters worse, because the shouting now leached into the night time. On the GP's recommendation I'd tried to reduce her Paroxetine. It'd made no difference to the noise, but her general agitation increased and the startle reflex that Mum exhibited in the mornings was more intense. So I'd reinstated the original dose of that particular drug.

Personally, I was going with the *'it may have become quite an established pattern in her life'* theory. In which case, I would have appreciated a drug that damped down the screaming and dispense with the psycho-babble, because I didn't see any way we were going to be able to improve the pattern of her life, or mine, by any other means.

And that, pretty much, was the message I relayed to the GP when I popped in to see him the following day. I'm not sure if I saw a wry smile flit across his face or not, but he put up no defence in favour of the psychologist's route to peace. He suggested that I take the direct approach and give the man a phone call to tell him how I felt about his suggestions, that way I could get my point across without any more misunderstandings.

Needless to say, I didn't make that phone call immediately, fear of man was the main reason. I had to be in a calm, assertive frame of mind to be able to present my case without getting rattled. That wasn't going to happen anytime soon.

* * *

My son was home from university and staying with his dad. I could put Ray out of my mind when Jake wasn't around to remind me of his father's existence. Jake said that there was evidence that Ray and his on/off girlfriend were now an item.

He'd been told, by a friend of his, that Penny had left her husband and was now living in a bungalow in the same close where my mother had resided, near to Ray's house. He told me about lengthy telephone calls that took place in the evenings in the privacy of Ray's bedroom and that the lounge had been re-vamped with a sense of style that would be alien to his father. Jake also knew that Ray was going to the Bristol International Balloon Fiesta.

He pointed out that his father was staying in a hotel, instead of with his

136

sister, who lived not far away in Bath. I had to admit that was definitely out of character, Ray never wandered far from the local pubs and spending money on a hotel in Bristol was off the gauge. Jake was sure his father and Penny were going together.

We were legally separated. There was nothing to be gained, financially, in getting a divorce, except closure and confirmation that this on/off affair of Ray's wasn't paranoia on my part, but the reason he'd been such a malicious husband for the last thirteen years of our relationship. I wanted to know, yet I didn't. Part of me didn't want to be involved in any of this.

I brooded on it, a pointless pastime unless I was able to do anything. I had a sudden germ of an idea, born from the impotence of not knowing for definite whether my husband was an adulterer or not. Ray was going to Bristol on the Thursday, if Penny was with him, she wouldn't be at work. I rang her place of employment on Thursday. It was a tourist information office, so staff there were used to taking calls all day. A woman answered. Not Penny.

'Hi could I speak to Penny B please?'

A business-like voice on my part, I'd done seven years on the reception desk at the district council offices, I knew the form.

'I'm sorry, Penny's on leave until Tuesday, can I help?'

'Oh what a fool I am, she was going to Bristol this weekend wasn't she?'

'Yes, to the Balloon Fiesta and it looks as if it will be a lovely weekend.'

'I've never been, but I should think if the weather's right it must be a spectacular sight. I'll give Penny a ring when she gets back. Thank you for your help, bye.'

That conversation didn't prove that they were together, but the weight of evidence was beginning to stack up. I could only get a divorce if they were committing adultery, catching them in bed together would have been conclusive evidence, but how likely was that scenario? Failing that, being together under the same roof overnight would suffice. I'd have to be patient. Ray would show his hand eventually. I was guessing that there were quite a few overnight stays while Jake was safely ensconced in Glamorgan. Jake had been home since early July and not due to go back until mid-September. Lust will out.

***

The screams continued unabated. I could tolerate it at a distance but when I was performing up close and personal tasks for Joan and she continued to scream in my space, her tongue protruding from her screwed up face, I could get to the point where I felt capable of doing almost anything to stop the noise. Many times I had to throw a blanket over her state of undress and walk out of the room. I wasn't prepared to risk imprisonment for murder.

On one particular day when she screamed from immediately after breakfast until 5pm with time out for lunch, I actually clamped my hand over her mouth and yelled at her.

'Shut up!'

Appalled at what I'd done, I ran into the garden, as far away from the source of my assault as I dared venture. How could I have done that? She was helpless and not responsible, but in that moment I'd felt the bile of hatred in my throat and the breathless pain of pent up anger in my chest. Danger signals I couldn't ignore. I needed to make that phone call to the psychologist and plead for a drug that would work.

After a prolonged time-out session of diaphragmatic breathing, I felt calmer and more able to cope. It was too late to phone the hospital, but I resolved to do it the next day. Joan remained unsettled and noisy, though the screaming had reduced to shouting, which was bearable.

***

Mum was put to bed a little later than usual, and when I went in to give her a drink and settle her for the night at about 9pm, she had quietened down but was still not asleep. The pump for the airwave mattress appeared excessively noisy. I reflected that even I'd have difficulty sleeping through that racket.

I went in again at 1am to change and turn her onto her other side. It took me a few seconds to register that there was now no noise in her bedroom. The pump had stopped working and the mattress was slowly deflating. My mother was virtually lying on the metal frame of the bed with just the ridged, airless mattress between her and excruciating discomfort. At that point, I wanted to throw in the towel, but that wasn't an option.

By the time I'd rolled Mum to get the hoist sling underneath her, the increased movement had totally flattened the mattress. I used the hoist to transfer her into the small armchair in the corner of her bedroom. I removed the now useless lump of rubber, then dragged the mattress off the spare bed. I had to work quickly, Mum wasn't safe in normal chairs, she would slide off them. I kept her attached to the hoist to reduce her movement. I slung the spare mattress on the bed, covered it with a duvet to soften it, then topped the whole lot with a mattress protector, sheet and absorbent bed pad. That done, I hoisted Mum back into bed, changed her, gave her a drink and turned her onto her left side. My mother, unbelievably, remained quiet and serene throughout the whole procedure. Ungraciously I thought, *If this is the kind of stimulation it takes to quieten you down, Mother, the psychologist can take a running jump off Hartland Point, because I'm not playing this game!*

I made it to bed by 3am and sunk into a deep sleep until nearly 9am. Mum didn't stir, even though I went into her in a panic, having overslept. I should have been turning her every four hours now she wasn't on an airwave mattress. She was still asleep, so I left her until I'd drunk coffee and planned my phone calls to the local hospital about the mattress and district hospital about the screaming.

The local hospital had just had an airwave mattress returned as no longer required, but, as yet, it hadn't been checked and cleaned so wouldn't be available until the next day. I supposed it was fortunate that there was one available at all as it was a game of chance. I accepted gratefully, promising that I would have the present one bagged up and ready to swap.

The second phone call was a little more complicated. I had to get my desperation across without seeming as if I couldn't cope at all, not an easy mix. The psychologist was sympathetic, but said he wanted to admit Joan into hospital for assessment and treatment.

I knew he was relatively new to Devon (I was beginning to suspect also new to the job) and obviously had no idea how unlikely that was, where people with advanced dementia, like my mother, were concerned.

'With respect,' I said. 'I don't think you'll find anywhere prepared to take her. Dementia patients always fare badly in hospital, the staff aren't trained and don't have the time to deal with their special needs. I don't think I'd be prepared to put my mother through that, even if you found somewhere, but I doubt if you will.'

I think I heard him bristle a little. He promised he'd ring again when he'd made enquiries.

***

On the 11th August, Jodi was giving me an afternoon and evening off so I could attend my niece's wedding in Torrington. Jake and his girlfriend also had an invitation and so did Ray, though not, I understood, his significant other, which I hoped would guarantee that Ray wouldn't make an appearance. It was going to be a church wedding and as I don't do church anything, weddings included, I waited outside, taking the photographs that nobody else got.

Charlotte paused, just before going into the church. For the benefit of my camera and to the amusement of the wedding groupies gathered together to view the bride, she raised her full and flowing dress to reveal her fancy footwear. Brand new blue trainers. An inspired combination of the practical and the superstitious.

I was given to understand that the service went without a hitch. Nobody fainted at the altar and the groom didn't forget the ring. The only glitch was that the vicar, semi-retired and maybe out of practice, forgot to ask 'Who gives this woman…?' It was to be Bob's starring role and it was a non-event. I supposed that the marriage was still legal.

The final hymn or song, not sure which heading it came under, nearly took the roof off the church. It was a rugby anthem sung by a congregation that were virtually all players and supporters of various rugby union teams.

The wedding line-up in the official photograph made me look old and more overweight than I'd ever been in my life, another reason to be relieved that Ray hadn't put in an appearance. I'd never considered myself to be a beauty, but at one time I could have held my own. Now I'd look like the ugly sister in comparison with Penny, who'd always maintained her smouldering good looks. I wondered what the attraction was on her part. Ray was eleven years her senior, certainly no looker, had a dicky heart and a drink problem. Not exactly catch of the year, yet I still didn't want him seeing me looking like a total frump. What complicated creatures we are.

By mid-August, Ray and Penny's relationship, a covert romance spanning twenty-five years or more was out in the open. Jake was expected to accept her as his new best friend. Knowing the misery this woman had brought to our home, his parents' marriage and to Jake, he wasn't prepared to make her welcome in the place that he still called home. What his father did was his father's business, but Jake made it clear that he didn't like Penny or, for that matter, her three sons. They'd already started seeking Jake out for veiled threats and abuse when the word was fed back to them about Jake's lack of cooperation. If Penny was in the house, he wasn't going to be there to play happy families.

It was during this revelation that I really broke the Golden Rule, big time. Thou shalt not bad mouth your spouse to your child. It transpired that Jake was under no illusion about his dad, but didn't want to get caught in the crossfire and that's just what I drew him into, by venting feelings that I'd bottled up for years. I felt terrible. That woman would, no doubt, have my son eating out of her hand before long. She seemed to have that effect on men, though tellingly, was universally disliked by women, none more than me.

Ray had reacted to this situation with his usual sensitivity and admirable maturity and refused to speak to Jake at all. Nobody can have an opinion that conflicts with Ray's without paying the price. Jake had learnt how to deal with his father, though I'm not sure he was prepared for the drunken punch Ray threw at him outside a pub in Bideford. That must have dealt an emotional blow which would have hurt far more than any physical one.

By reverting to non-opinionated mode, Jake signalled submission without actually submitting. Thus normal surface serenity was restored, but of course, the subject had been struck off the list of topics for conversation or discussion. Jake still refused to have anything to do with the girlfriend.

The relationship between Jake and his father was one they'd have to sort out for themselves but I had the strong feeling that Ray would be the loser, long term. The upside, if there was one, was that I could now convert my judicial separation into a divorce, but now I could, I suddenly wasn't in any hurry. Just knowing I was free to do it was enough for the time being.

Chapter Twenty-Two

The psychologist rang me back. I'd been right, hospitalisation for Mum wasn't feasible. He wanted to prescribe a drug called Risperdal, a newer antipsychotic, not normally used with dementia patients. He'd have liked her to have been in hospital when she began taking it, in case there were any adverse reactions, but that option wasn't available to him. I would have to administer the drug at home.

She was due to go for a week's respite care on the twelfth of September and Jodi was getting married on the eighth. I gave Mum her first dose of Risperdal on the morning of the wedding. I got her up and dressed and packed into the van to fulfil my promise to be outside the registry office when Jodi and Paul emerged as a married couple.

By the time we arrived at the venue, my mother was extremely drowsy. When Jodi and Sharnie, in bridesmaid regalia, came over to give her a kiss, she had begun to slump over the side of the wheelchair. We stayed until the bridal party had moved on to the reception. By then my mother was almost comatose and I was seriously concerned that I'd overdosed her.

When we got back home I double-checked the prescription. I'd given her the correct amount but, of course, I'd forgotten the unwritten rule. Always, always when giving a new course of medication to the elderly, begin with a lower dose that the prescription specifies and work upwards, or not, depending on results. I was so desperate to stop the screaming, I'd effectively overdosed her.

Mum was out of it for the entire afternoon and well into the evening, not rousable at all. The silence was deafening and totally unnerved me. I was glued to her, taking observations every fifteen minutes, scared to death that she was going to die on me, due to the psychologist's inexperience and my negligence and over-enthusiasm for peace. This, of course, was precisely the reason he'd wanted to administer the drug in hospital.

I needn't have worried. The following day she was back with me, albeit a lot quieter, but then that was the point of the medication. However, I did reduce the dose by a half and intended keeping it at that until she came back from respite care.

The respite week started on the Wednesday and I had a mountain of ironing to get through before I could pack her suitcase. Because of the washing she managed to generate in a single day, I'd purchased a tumble dryer (best invention ever, after chocolate). As Mum's clothes were of the stretchy, fleecy variety, they rarely required ironing, they came out of the drier soft, warm and ready to wear.

With all the kerfuffle at the weekend, I'd forgotten the load I'd put into the dryer until I went to insert freshly washed clothes. The sheets, towels and clothes had taken on grunge mode, indelibly creased. I toyed with the idea of putting them through a rinse cycle and tumble-drying them again, but the mean streak in me said 'no' to the extra electricity. I'd done the crime, now I had to put in the time.

Mum was still subdued as a result of the Risperdal. It was wonderful not to have to endure the constant shouting and screaming, but I didn't want a chemical cosh that would reduce her to a zombie. At the moment, on just half the recommended dose, she was drowsy and not anywhere near as alert as she had been. Maybe she was still suffering the after effects of the overdose or maybe this was the choice, zombie or banshee. I decided to leave things as they were until she got back from respite care.

I set up the ironing board in the lounge, in front of the television. It was a luxury. I didn't usually have the opportunity during the day to watch TV and was too exhausted at night to be bothered.

The TV programme that should have been on, wasn't, instead the screen came to life with a man sky-diving from a high rise building, only he wasn't sky-diving, he was falling and there was smoke billowing out from the disabled building. For a second or two I thought I was in the middle of a film. The commentator was shouting his despair above the noise of screams and sirens, his voice choked with horror and disbelief. I couldn't take in that what I was witnessing through the eye of the camera, was happening in real time in New York. I watched, transfixed, as the second plane struck the south tower of the World Trade Centre. The commentator was still focused on possible freak accidents. Did anyone really believe that? It seemed that everyone who witnessed the horror and heartbreak as these events unfolded, would be joined together by the single thought, if this can happen here, in the USA, there's nowhere in the world that's safe anymore. We'd witnessed a pivotal moment in history that would trigger unspeakable consequences.

***

The front garden had to be rejigged. I dug deep into limited energy resources to achieve the makeover in my week's break. I also needed to be doing physical work to counteract the negative thought processes.

I dug up an unidentifiable bush that'd been planted in the centre of the lawn. It not only obscured vision up the road when reversing out of the drive, but was also an obstruction to mowing the grass. I spared the rowan tree, simply because it was too big to grapple with. It'd made its home right next to the public footpath, so required regular pruning to prevent the decapitation of passing pedestrians. The berries of the rowan, although an attractive autumnal feature on the tree and excellent for wildlife, were a pain to clear up from the ground and baby rowan trees grew like weeds.

Both back and front gardens had taken on a cared-for look but the back garden still needed work. One of the last jobs, which required more muscle power than I possessed, had been completed by Jake, Tim and Tim's dad's people-carrier. It entailed the removal of bags of excavated rubble to be transported to the council's refuse tip. With that cleared, I could complete the groundwork, ready for planting in the spring.

On reflection it was almost inconceivable that I'd planned that far ahead. Dr A had, at one time, expressed the view that Joan was unlikely to survive the first twenty-four hours if we put her through the stress of moving from Huesneath Moor, but she was still here, very much alive and kicking. She'd gained weight, was eating well, her skin was flawless and she was escaping the confines of home on an almost daily basis. Now, if I could just solve the inappropriate vocalisation dilemma, we'd be on a roll.

***

I also took advantage of my week off to catch up on phone calls to people I wanted to stay in contact with. One of those favoured few was my cousin, Pam. My aunt Joan had died about a year before I took Mum out of HM. She'd spent her last month or so in hospital, with Pam going in every day to feed her and give her the general care that the hospital staff seemed incapable of providing. It was only after her mum had died that Pam understood that her mother had likely been an early victim of the Liverpool Care Pathway and that the staff had been implementing the misinterpreted ethics of this form of palliative care.

The LCP was an approach to the palliative care of terminally ill cancer patients, developed at the Marie Curie Hospital, Liverpool and the Royal Liverpool University Hospital in the late 1990s. It was supposed to mean that doctors could stop treatment if it would result in a more comfortable death, or withdraw food and drink if patients declined it.

The LCP was supposed to ensure that terminal patients in their last weeks/days/hours of life would receive a standard of care that would minimise pain, discomfort and distress given with kindness, compassion and dignity.

Government ministers announced in the summer of 2013 that the LCP would be phased out following a government commissioned review which uncovered evidence of abuse, including patients being unnecessarily sedated and denied food and water.

The review made forty-four recommendations, including the phasing out of LCP as individual care plans for the dying are brought in. Only senior clinicians will make the decision to give end of life care, along with the healthcare team. There must be no incentive payments to hospitals to put patients on end of life care, as occurred with the LCP. The payment had been intended to provide encouragement to adopt best practice, but had been interpreted as payments to speed up patients' demise.

I don't think there is much doubt in the minds of people who have worked in the field of care giving, especially of the elderly with dementia, that the LCP was used, in some cases, as a form of euthanasia.

Pam and her husband, Ken had looked after Pam's mum at home for five years and since her mother's death, Pam had suffered one illness after another. She didn't say, but I thought that she'd become so exhausted in her role as carer, that her immune system was now on the floor, hence the state she was in now.

Pam had some obscure virus that had affected her lungs and after a biopsy had shown no sinister cause, she'd been left to get on with it. Further investigation by Pam disclosed that it could have been an adverse reaction to shellfish additives in a naturopath's preparation for arthritis. Now she was having osteopathic treatment for her back and they'd managed to damage her ribcage or some cartilage in her sternum. Whichever it was, she was in a great deal of pain. Personally, I thought I recognised the symptoms of depression mixed up in all this.

***

My mother returned from respite care with her eyes glued shut, diarrhoea and dehydration. I had that same sinking feeling that I couldn't do this again, but I needed the break. In fact I'd thought, during her absence, of asking Bob if we could afford to extend respite to two weeks at a time. I despaired at Mum's condition when she returned home and decided to shelve that idea for the time being.

It took a few days for her to fully recover before I could make a proper assessment of the effects of Risperdal. It soon became apparent that half the prescribed amount wasn't enough. I gradually increased the drug until she was taking the full dose. Nothing. Risperdal was doing nothing. "The Scream" was back. I'm not sure if I didn't glimpse a glint of triumph in Joan's eyes, probably not, but it was beginning to seem like a personal vendetta on her part. At a loss to know what to do next, I did nothing, just kept hoping that Risperdal would work the next day.

***

The events of August and September, adultery, wedding, terrorism, betrayal, plus Jake returning to Glamorgan, had a profoundly depressing effect. Jake had been back quite often during his first year at university, mainly because his girlfriend was still in Bideford. Now Harriet was joining him in Glamorgan as she embarked on her first year in higher education.

Given the present circumstances, I couldn't see him coming home very often, if at all. Virtually all his close friends were at different universities scattered throughout the country except one close friend, Simon, who'd started at the same university with Jake but had chosen to leave. He'd been homesick and didn't enjoy the experience and bravely, I thought, made the decision that it wasn't for him and came home.

Jake had a clutch of very close friends and he worked at keeping the group in touch with each other. He arranged get-togethers and went the extra mile to nurture the relationships. He'd worked through the summer holidays to accrue funds to bolster the coming academic year. Living had been cheap in Devon because he'd stayed at home during the holidays, but if Penny moved in, I didn't see him returning there at Christmas. Still, there was always a spare room here which he'd utilised a couple of times during the summer when the atmosphere at home had become particularly antagonistic and intolerable.

Jake had left on an uneasy truce. Word of his perceived treachery in failing to accept Penny had filtered to his aunt, Ray's sister, the only one of Ray's relatives who remained in regular contact with Ray or Jake. Now she wouldn't speak to her nephew, preferring to believe her brother's version of events, whatever that was.

Tessa, my Sunday care worker, was going through a bad time in her life too. Her husband had walked out on her. She was devastated. He was ten years younger than her, but it'd seemed a solid relationship. Tessa had no inkling that there was someone else in his life. I'd never met him, but had seen him working at a local supermarket. He always struck me as a slightly awkward, socially inept type, but it's not easy to judge by the way a man stacks shelves.

Tessa licked her wounds for a few weeks, with tears and recriminations which I absorbed with empathy, having bought the T-shirt. Then she went slightly crazy and took to clubbing on Friday and Saturday nights. I admit, I'd never experienced the delights of this particular activity so I was certainly no expert but it seemed inappropriate and counter-productive as a pay-back tactic which I assumed was the motive behind behaviour which screamed lack of self respect.

Clubbing, for Tessa, entailed getting drunk and having sexual intercourse with anyone capable of making the right moves. While I knew this all came from pain and heartbreak, I really didn't want the detailed account she felt compelled to impart each week.

It was with a profound sense of relief that I accepted her resignation in early December. The reason given was that she couldn't tolerate Joan's screaming. I guess it didn't mix well with the Sunday hangover.

I advertised immediately for a replacement, but this close to Christmas everyone, it seemed, was totally focused on the festive season, I didn't hold out much hope. Jodi stepped into the breach and covered every other Sunday when she could. I was very grateful, but knew it wasn't a satisfactory arrangement for either of us.

***

Mum developed a slight sniffle just before Christmas and by the 23rd she was comatose. I couldn't rouse her at all. I panicked. The thought of Christmas looming with three days flying solo was absolutely fine with me, if my mother had been her usual stroppy self, but now she looked as if she was dying. I rang the surgery for a home visit.

Mum's GP was on leave and it was a young doctor who arrived. He was fairly new to the practice and my heart sank a little, but I needn't have worried. He reassured me that I'd done the right thing by calling him out. He sounded her chest, pneumonia being an obvious possibility, but her chest was clear. He ran a finger along the soles of her feet and lightly touched her eyeball to provoke a reaction. There wasn't one. He explained, in a very gentle way, that he could admit her into hospital, but she was getting far better care here.

He didn't know what was wrong. With dementia patients, in the end stage of the disease, it was sometimes very difficult to know what was going on internally without invasive tests. Would I really want to put Joan through that?

'We never know, what part of the brain is going to be destroyed next,' he said, 'but you have to be prepared for what may come in the future if she recovers from this. For example, if her swallow reflex goes, will you want Joan to be fed through a tube directly into her stomach, or palliative care to keep her comfortable and pain free?'

These were all aspects of the end of life process that I was familiar with. I'd already made my decisions on Mum's behalf when I took on this role as carer. Those decisions still held good. I'd needed to be re-focused. I'd momentarily lost sight of the value of quality of life, rather than life for life's sake. It was all too easy to succumb to the ambush of sentiment and the desire to be seen as a competent carer.

The doctor replaced his stethoscope in his bag and prepared to leave.

'It'll be kinder to your mother if she can stay in her own home, but only you know if you can take what comes. There's no shame in saying that you don't think you can accept the responsibility. What I can tell you is, you're doing a great job and you're doing all that can be done and more. Do you understand where I'm coming from?'

I did. I'd simply needed reminding that my mother was at the end stage of her life. It was easy to accept the status quo as being, if not normal, then a situation that would go on for years unaltered. The facts were, my mother had come out of a nursing home with a diagnosis of end stage dementia and a prognosis of weeks, rather than months of life left. Good care had extended that life span, but it hadn't altered the diagnosis and the end could come at any time. Maybe today was the day.

The doctor gave me a bottle of Oramorph, in case Mum became distressed. He left me in no doubt that I was to expect the worst. Having had the pep talk, my confidence had been renewed. I could cope, after all I'd been through this many times before as a care worker. I had all the kit I would require, I'd even bought a pretty nightdress, to lay Mum out in.

***

My mother was unconscious for forty-eight hours, then gradually woke up and by Boxing Day was virtually back to normal. When Jodi came in on the 27th it was very difficult to convey that I'd seriously expected her to be out of a job by now.

Two days before the start of the New Year, I had a phone call from a lady called Heather. She'd seen my advert in the paper and wondered if the job had been taken. I tried to curb the impulse to sound too desperate and arranged an interview for the next day. Heather had worked as a home carer, on and off, plus other jobs that fitted around rearing two boys. Her husband was a lot older than her and found our winters difficult to cope with, so would escape to their home in Cyprus for the winter months. Meanwhile Heather, who wanted her boys to be educated in Britain, rented a house here. A complicated life, entangled even further because her youngest son was being targeted by a bunch of bullies from the school that he attended.

I could relate to that because Jake had also been bullied, though this had happened in primary school. Eventually, I took action as the school seemed incapable of doing anything constructive even though some of the episodes of bullying had happened in the classroom, right under the nose of the class teacher. I'd been up to the school many times to ask for help to make it stop. The final straw came when they waylaid my son on his way to a school fund-raising event and relieved him of his spending money.

I rang the mother of the ringleader and we all got together at her house, me, Jake, the Little Thug and his parents. I say Little Thug, because he was very small in stature (which may have been at the core of the problem) but big on attitude and, as I recall, an excellent artist and skate boarder. In the style of all the best criminal minds, he never got his hands dirty, he simply made the bullets. Little Thug had a henchman, a much bigger kid, in size rather than brain function, who did all the damage. It transpired that this lad was himself being bullied at home by a stepfather.

The meeting of minds had been successful. I let Jake put his own case across and Little Thug's parents encouraged their son to explain why he was masterminding criminal activities. It was all unexpectedly civilised, and the bullying that Jake had endured for the best part of four years, stopped. In fact, Jake and Little Thug became, if not best buddies, friends, when both entered secondary education. The henchman had, by then, moved away and I remained on friendly terms with Little Thug's mum.

Heather was pleased to step into the breach and didn't appear too put off by my mother's expert ability at breaking the sound barrier, a skill which was beginning to gain momentum again now that she'd recovered from her mystery illness. Mum appeared to have developed an added disability. Now, she pouched food in her cheeks like a hamster and choked more easily than before. We had to clear the debris from her mouth with swabs after every meal to minimise the risk.

By the end of January I was going stir crazy. The weather wasn't conducive to going out anywhere and being trapped indoors 24/7 with "The Scream" wore me down and wound me up, simultaneously. The Risperdal was doing absolutely nothing, as far as I could tell.

One afternoon, in desperation, I rang the clinical psychologist on his direct line. I'd given the drug a fair trial, I'd heard nothing from him in the interim period and despaired of ever being a participant of the talked about team approach. I was tired, angry and about to give this man my uncensored verdict on Risperdal, only he wasn't there.

An older man, judging by the voice, answered the phone. He gave me his name, but my brain was re-booting at the time and I didn't take it in, but the important fact was he was a clinical psychologist and head of the department. A talk with the organ grinder, rather than the monkey, sounded good to me.

I explained the problem from the beginning. He listened to me and to Joan, screaming fit to burst, in the background.

'How on earth do you manage to stay sane with that noise going on?'

Good question.

'I'm not and I'm afraid of what I might do to her if it goes on for much longer.'

He was sympathetic, but I no longer wanted sympathy, I wanted action and I wanted it now. And that was the heartfelt desire I conveyed to my new ally.

'I'm going to prescribe a drug called Largactyl,' he said. 'This isn't a new drug, it's been around since the fifties, which means it's been tried and tested and it will work.'

Brave words. By then I was clutching at straws while drowning but I really wanted to believe him.

Within the week Risperdal had been returned to the pharmacy and Largactil had been collected and administered. I wasn't holding my breath, but when peace descended at 42 Water Park Road, I felt the tension leave my shoulders. Largactyl did work! It was as if someone had replaced the evil twin with her calm, benevolent sister. The drug didn't appear to make Mum drowsy, it simply turned off the hollering. It was wonderful. Caring for my mother became a pleasure rather than a thankless chore. It wasn't until then that I realised just how stressed and depressed I'd become.

Chapter Twenty-Three

The rest of the winter and spring was quiet, with an atmosphere of holistic calm. I was able to learn more about my mother, as the person she was now. For example, I discovered that she had distinct likes and dislikes about the music that was played at home. Unfortunately, her likes weren't often on the same wavelength as mine.

When I moved out of the marital home and was first on my own, I had a stab at sequence ballroom dancing. Some friends had formed their own club and invited me along. I can't say that I really enjoyed it. Ballroom dancing is fine with a male partner, but I wasn't keen on dancing with another woman. As there was a shortage of men, there was little option.

David Last was an organist, not the church type, but these electronic gadgets that can become any instrument you like at the touch of a button. He came and played for the club on several occasions which was a refreshing change from taped music. Though it wasn't my kind of music, then or now, I was persuaded to buy one of his cassette tapes so I could practise the "Mayfair Quickstep" and the "Sally Ann Cha Cha" in the privacy of my own home. The vain hope was that it might help me to move in sequence or, at least, in the same general direction and rhythm as the other dancers. That never happened and I abandoned sequence dancing as a lost cause.

The tape, however, was still in my possession and Mum had loved ballroom dancing. The tunes on the tape had very distinctive rhythms and I presumed that, for anyone who was au fait with ballroom dancing, it would be obvious if David was playing a foxtrot or a samba.

Would it evoke in her memories of past times or awaken an internal rhythm to which she could relate? She remained very quiet throughout the entire tape but her foot was bobbing, seemingly to a beat. Coincidence? I wasn't absolutely sure, but the foot movement stopped when the music ceased. I asked my sequence ballroom friends if they could procure me a different tape, which they were happy to provide. That gave me an hour's worth of David Last, which appeared to be fine with my mother, but I was suffering.

I was now on a mission to extend the repertoire. I tried music from my collection to establish if we had more in common than I'd thought. Using the toe-bobbing measurement, I had to discount most of my taste in music, except for "The Carpenters" and a random country and western compilation CD. Perhaps not so random, when I stopped to think about it. Dad had given me a home-recorded cassette tape of the country and western CD and I'd liked it enough to buy a better recording. My father had a large collection of cassette tapes, nearly all home recordings of radio programmes, borrowed CDs and vinyl records. Both "The Carpenters" cassette and the country and western music had entered my collection via my father.

On one of our outings to Atlantic Village, we went into a shop where you could buy retro gear. Jewellery boxes with ballerinas that twirled to a tune when the lids were lifted, space hoppers, spinning tops and CDs with old songs going back to the war years. I bought two CDs, the "Andrews Sisters" and "Chas and Dave". The latter was an unlikely choice on the face of it, but in the late seventies, the whole family had been to see "Chas and Dave" singing live in a London pub. Their music had been a bonding factor at family gatherings throughout the intervening years.

This selection of music provided the core of my mother's list of toe-bobbing entertainment. I continued to experiment with other genres, with some success, but always gravitated back to the same tried and tested few.

We had Radio Devon on in the mornings until I'd completed Mum's ablutions and moved out of the bedroom. Radio Devon was more for my benefit than hers. I liked Judi Spiers, she made me laugh out loud and that didn't happen too often. I enjoyed the banter and the interaction with listeners. It was easy listening as I worked my way through the morning routine. Judi often read out poetry or observational pieces sent in by listeners, and I pondered about the possibility of sending a poem into the show. The problem was, I didn't really want to attach my name to anything. I wrote a poem about looking after Mum, signed it "A Carer" and sent it in with a request for Celine Dion's "Think Twice".

To my unexpected delight it was read out on air. Judi said, 'We don't usually read out items that have been sent in anonymously (the A Carer pseudonym hadn't fooled her then) but as it's Carer's Week (I didn't know we had a week) and the nature of the poem is so poignant and relevant, I'm going to make an exception and read it.'

She left out one verse as I recall, which mentioned defecation, but I thought she recited it with just the right tone. It was followed by my Celine request, which I never got to hear because the phone rang. It was Kathy, my work colleague from the residential home, who helped me compile my care plan and who'd hoped to take her own mother into her care when the hospital had stabilised her.

Kathy had recognised the poem as fitting my profile and thought I might have been the author. So much for remaining totally unattached to this literary feat. We chatted for a while. She'd looked after her mum for a few months, up until she died without ever regaining any, except the very basic, faculties. Still, Kathy was thankful that she'd been in a position to give her the best palliative care possible for those last weeks.

I received another phone call later in the day from a friend who'd also heard the programme. She had an inkling that it might have been my handiwork. She said it'd made her cry. I don't know if that was my intention, it was more of a cathartic outpouring on my part.

TO ALL HOME CARERS — A MUCH UNDERVALUED WORKFORCE

I think of myself as a single mother,
why? Because I have no significant other.
My babe is my mum, with Alzheimer's, I'm told.
She functions at maybe four months old.

Joan's body is useless and so is her brain,
though thankfully there isn't much pain.
She was in a home, but the care was so bad
and in the end I got really mad.

Nothing I said made a difference you see.
To add insult to injury, Mum paid her own fee.
She went in walking, but with violent intent,
as time went by her speech and legs went.

Joan spent her days in a cold room,
always shouting, morning, night and noon.
No home would have her because of the noise,
though it couldn't be said we were spoilt for choice.

My marriage was over, my son fully grown,
my circumstance changed, I was now on my own.
Could I take her on? I wasn't a nurse,
but I'd worked as a carer, so first things first.

The doctor said. 'No, she won't last the pace.'
'Better that, I said, 'than the abuse in that place.'
He agreed that all I said was true.
He said. 'Okay, but you must think this through.'

To take on Joan's care was a major decision,
had to be planned with military precision.
Sixteen months she's been living with me.
The experts were wrong, though I doubt they'd agree.

Frankly, I hope that each day is her last.
Quality of life is diminishing fast.
Human life's become cheap that's the point to be made,
a throwaway mindset, it's of this I'm afraid.

Not everyone is in my position,
to care for a loved one in such a frail condition.
I have no political stance to pursue,
but better care for our elderly is long overdue.

Joan was just a wife and a mother,
gave life to me and my younger brother.
Joan could be you, or you, or you.
Once it's here, it's too late to change your point of view.

***

Jake had returned home at Christmas though he didn't stay with his dad. Relations there were still very volatile. Ray spent more time with Penny's sons than his own. Ray's sister still wasn't speaking to Jake, the poison having been well and truly administered. Jake was stoical about it all but reluctant to discuss it with me though the injustice must have hurt.

He split his living arrangements between Harriet's home, Simon's settee and my spare room. I'd doubted whether he would come back at all, but Harriet obviously wanted to because she had close family ties in Bideford and many of Jake's friends came home for the Christmas and New Year celebrations.

Ray was spending money wildly to meet the requirements of his girlfriend. Meals out often and holidays abroad. This rankled with me, I'd rather not have known. He'd been so tight fisted with money when we'd been together, not just towards me, but with Jake as well. Now, he was throwing money at this hard-faced piece of work like there was no tomorrow.

The Easter holidays of 2002 brought more heartbreak. One of Jake's group of close friends was killed in a freak motorbike accident. He was riding pillion when the bike went out of control along the A39 near Clovelly. The camber of the road was in question, but no one really knew the cause. The biker sustained minor injuries, but Matt died at the scene. His parents had been riding behind him on another bike and were both with him. There was no obvious external injury, but Matt's life ended at the roadside.

Jake was asked if he'd be a bearer at the funeral. Naturally he said yes, but it must have been an incredibly emotional and harrowing role to fulfil. It devastated the group of friends. At that age you think you're invincible, now they were forced to realise that in the blink of an eye your life can be over. Jake didn't show much emotion, but neither did he want to talk about it. How Matt's parents coped, I couldn't begin to imagine.

At the end of April, Penny left Ray, for reasons unknown, although Ray blamed Jake. I don't suppose for one moment that Ray thought of himself as being in any way to blame. His drink problem always transformed him into a nasty individual. His lack of control over his drinking was never going to be reined in by love or lust. In my experience, most alcoholics are rarely responsive in a positive way to external events. When confronted with the prospect of achieving something better, Ray would only manage to hold his dependency in check for a limited period, before he sabotaged his life. If he'd ever been on the wagon, he'd now fallen off without dignity.

I personally never thought that Penny had been in love with Ray. She was, however, a woman who couldn't be without a man in her life. Although I didn't blame her for not wanting to remain with the Jekyll and Hyde personality that was my husband, I could almost guarantee that she would have somebody else waiting in the wings before she made her decision to part company with Ray and Ray's money. Until she showed her hand, Jake made a convenient, if implausible, scapegoat for them both.

***

Five months into the realms of peace induced by Largactyl, Mum was still responding well to this drug. There was a little breakthrough shouting as she developed a tolerance to it, but it was at a manageable level, nothing like the screaming of the previous year. With the arrival of better weather we were able to escape the confines of the bungalow and resume our afternoon outings. Our haunts remained the same, Victoria Park still being high on the list as an outside venue. It wasn't scenery that held any appeal for my mother, it was people, more specifically, children. Any place where there were kids was okay with her.

We were well into the second year of looking after Mum at home. Life had fallen into an inevitable pattern and her condition appeared stable. There was deterioration, but it was slow. We overcame each obstacle, almost without noticing that it was another marker, pointing towards the end of her life.

Heather was a competent carer and now a friend. I was pleased that she was onboard, knowing that, like Jodi, she would step into the breach, over and above her set hours whenever she could. Her youngest boy sometimes, but rarely, came with her. Now in his teens, he was reluctant to be stuck here with his mother and a demented old lady and who could blame him.

Sharnie was still on board as an unpaid carer. She took over a parental role with Mum. Sharnie was one of the few individuals who she responded to with facial expressions. I have a photograph of Sharnie posing with her arms wrapped around my mother's neck. Mum's face is expressing mock distaste at this embrace, but she loved it, Sharnie was her best buddy. One problem that was looming on the horizon, was inadvertently caused by Sharnie. She would soon be starting school. Jodi and I had discussed it, but we were having difficulty seeing a way around the impact this would have on the hours that Jodi worked. I was trying to reconcile myself to having my own free time curtailed.

Respite care was set at one week in every three months. Although Mum was much easier to care for now that the screaming had stopped, it was becoming increasingly hard physically and the lack of spontaneity in my life and sense of entrapment was sometimes difficult to cope with. I couldn't just pop to the chemist to pick up a prescription because somebody had to be with her at all times. I roped my brother in for a spell of mother-sitting. He'd only called round, to touch base, on his way back home from work, but I needed antibiotics for yet another UTI that was causing Mum discomfort.

It was my fault, I was supposed to get the tablets on the Thursday, but had forgotten. It was now Friday. I'd resigned myself to being without until Jodi came in next week. I was in the middle of giving Mum her tea when Bob turned up. I handed him the dish of mashed banana and custard, with instructions about the words that would encourage Mum to open her mouth and the promise that I would only be ten minutes.

Thankfully, it wasn't any longer. When I returned, she was wearing more banana and custard than she'd consumed, her face was awash with the stuff. Bob was looking rueful but unrepentant. He'd used the magic words, but her mouth had refused to open.

'I told you I couldn't be hands-on,' he said.

***

I didn't have to wait too long before the real reason for Penny's departure became obvious. Jake found out through his contacts that Penny had found herself a younger model. Somebody else's husband, who'd left his wife and children to be with Penny. There was a thaw between Jake and his father and Ray's sister was speaking again. I was pleased for Jake, though felt he was owed an apology from both of them, which, of course, wasn't forthcoming.

Jake had finished university and armed with his degree was looking for work that matched his qualifications. In the interim, he worked for an agency and had secured a temporary job as a dustman. On the day of his graduation, Jodi took over the reins so that I could attend the presentation. Personally, I lacked appreciation for the plethora of university degrees that were available, unless they were a means to becoming a doctor or something equally beneficial to humanity. I would be far more impressed if I could find a qualified plumber when I needed one, but that sort of qualification seemed in short supply. Still, Jake had worked hard for his degree and I wanted to be there to see him receiving his diploma. Two problems, this shindig was in Bristol and Ray was going to be there.

Bob said he'd take me if I didn't mind that he'd be in his bus driver's uniform. I really didn't care if he turned up in a leopard print onesie as long as I got there, so we went together. It wasn't going to be easy, Bob still thought of himself as a friend of Ray's and how was I going to play it?

Rick, a friend of mine, whose wife had left him some years before, but for whom he still held a cathedral-sized candle, suggested that I went for stunning. Now, presentable I could do, at a push, but stunning was out of reach.

'Lose a bit of weight, buy a dress that flatters, get your hair done properly, not your usual home-hacked job and buy some killer heels,' Rick said.

He had a point. I'd totally let myself go. I couldn't aspire to stunning, but I could do better.

***

I was quietly pleased with the overall effect on the day. I'd managed to lose a few pounds, but went for a straight shift look anyway, the few pounds hadn't made that much of an impact. I was, however, sporting the professional haircut and the killer heels were on my feet, I just hoped I didn't have to walk too far.

Jake was waiting at a pre-arranged rendezvous. Bob had intended to stay in the car with his newspaper, but I needed the support, Red Bus uniform or not. I briefly met up with Jake, Harriet and Ray before we went in. I smiled graciously and hoped I managed to hide the shock I felt at seeing Ray again, for the first time in nearly five years. He'd shrunk, he looked old and his

154

teeth were in need of some serious attention, so why was I feeling so jittery?

We all trooped into the auditorium, Ray and Harriet went to sit in the gallery, while I chose to sit in the floor area of the auditorium, with Bob. I have to admit to a lurch of pride as Jake went up on stage to collect his diploma, tempered by sadness when the father of one of Jake's close associates, a friendship formed at university, received a diploma on behalf of his son. His child had died suddenly with a heart defect he'd unknowingly harboured all his short life.

Students and their families gathered in a huge marquee for celebratory drinks. Ray hung about on the periphery, while I threw myself into talking to all and sundry in an attempt to appear normal and unfazed. Inside I just wanted to cut and run. I noticed that Ray had disappeared. I asked Jake where he was.

'Outside,' he shrugged.

I felt guilty and I'd no idea why.

***

There was an official photographer's studio set up in one of the lecture rooms and I badgered Jake into agreeing to have a commemorative photo taken and to ask his father if he would agree to have a family photo done. Ray refused. Undeterred, I buoyantly insisted that I needed a photograph of Jake in his cap and gown, it was a parental right. Jake had a photo taken on his own and another with Harriet and me. I did momentarily think that I'd have liked one done with just the two of us, but not wanting to appear possessive, I let it go. I ordered copies, paid and returned to the marquee to collect my brother.

Bob was deep in conversation with Ray, but had the good grace to cease fraternising when he caught sight of me. I managed to say a light-hearted goodbye (at least that's what I was aiming for) to my husband, who merely nodded his head once in acknowledgement that he'd heard me. I wanted to run back to the sanctuary of the car, but the killer heels were living up to their description.

Weeks later, when the photographs arrived, I sent one of Jake to his father.

Chapter Twenty-Four

We'd reached 2003 and exhaustion had become my nemesis. When Jodi took over, I would escape to my room, to sleep or read, if my time wasn't allotted elsewhere. I had begun to feel that life was going on around me, but I was no longer part of it. A week's respite only scratched the surface as a period of recuperation and the journey was a trial for Mum now. It was too far and before she'd had time to recover, she had the journey home to contend with.

The respite care wasn't brilliant, but I'd tried to find somewhere else. A number of the nursing homes offered respite care, but none of them would consider fixed bookings, except the home I was using. I was stuck with the present arrangement, but needed longer. I was still weighing up the pros and cons, but the idea of the extra time off was very appealing.

Bob reassured me that there was more than enough money to fund the extra respite care, but baulked, in principal, at the idea of paying Jodi and Heather during the extra time that Mum would be away from home.

'That's the equivalent of eight weeks holiday a year. No care workers get that,' he said.

We weren't talking thousands of pounds here and both the girls were entitled to four weeks statutory holiday pay. As I pointed out, I didn't want to risk losing two good carers for the sake of the extra paid leave. I failed to mention to Bob that Jodi actually had nine weeks paid holiday. The extra was so she could have spare hours to use as and when she needed to. Now that Sharnie was at school, there would be the occasional crisis or school event that Jodi would need time for. The extra leave could make the difference between her being happy to remain as Mum's carer or feeling torn between the two roles. Sometimes it's prudent to keep your own counsel.

The anticipated problem of Sharnie starting school never materialised. Another mother, whose daughter went to the same school and who lived in Water Park Road, was happy to drop Sharnie off at the bungalow on the two afternoon shifts that Jodi worked.

***

With the autumn of 2003 came the news that Penny's boyfriend had left her and returned to his wife and children. Momentarily without a man, Penny turned her attention to the soft touch that was my husband.

'Surely he won't take her back?' my son said.

'I'm sure he will,' I replied, with certainty and sudden insight.

Ray had always been obsessed with this woman. She'd be free to come and go at will, and Ray would accept it, doubtless with protest, threats and promises, but he'd always take her back.

I could no longer perceive of any reason why I should remain married to Ray. For reasons best known to him, he hadn't instigated divorce proceedings, but I was now ready to cut the final ties. I made an appointment with the solicitor.

By this time, Jake was living with Harriet so it wasn't difficult to avoid his father's home. But needless to say, the relationship with Ray, fragile at best, was now being undermined again as Penny stalked her way back into Ray's life with claws sharpened for the kill. Now there was talk of the pair of them selling their respective homes and buying a house together. Jake was again subjected to threats from Penny's sons, because he refused to welcome her with open arms, which had the effect of pushing Jake further from reconciliation. It was a mess, with a predictable outcome.

***

In September 2003 Mum had two weeks respite care for the first time. The home didn't do much more damage in a fortnight than they'd managed to do in the previous respite periods of one week. She came home with glued-up eyes, nappy rash and weight loss as usual, plus the standard UTI that she always contracted during her time away from home. The UTI would trigger the "inappropriate vocalisation" which, under normal circumstances, was no longer a problem, but if Mum was sore, itchy and running a low grade fever with the infection there was every reason to shout.

The doctor and I had reached an unspoken understanding. As long as I didn't abuse the system, if I rang asking for antibiotics for a UTI, I got them without having to produce a urine sample which was almost impossible to provide. My mother hadn't actually seen a doctor since the home visit at Christmas 2001. I received the occasional visit from the community nurse, usually with a probationary nurse in tow. Mum provided a good teaching aid for the demonstration of end stage Alzheimer's disease.

In December, Mum had another two week respite break. When she returned home, I made the decision that she wouldn't be going again. Mum was now too frail to withstand the discomfort of the journey and the inadequate care at the home.

In the two weeks she'd been away, she had deteriorated. Her limbs were starting to contract upwards and inwards towards a foetal position. I hadn't noticed this was happening before she went away, but maybe the fortnight's gap enabled me see her condition through fresh and less exhausted eyes.

The community nurse suggested that physiotherapy might help reduce the rigidity of my mother's limbs. The physiotherapist showed me a range of exercises to be carried out on a daily basis to relax the tension in her limbs and neck. There would be no more trips out in the van, even the time sitting in her recliner was reduced to the mornings only. In bed, I was able to vary her position to a much greater extent than was possible in the chair.

Mum was still eating well, though her ability to open her bowels unaided, even after a suppository, was presenting a problem. As a care assistant, I'd never done a manual evacuation of the bowel, it was always a qualified nurse who'd carried out this intimate task. I'd been present to assist so I'd seen it done and also knew the inherent dangers.

It was a procedure that was only carried out when all else had failed. I was reluctant to ask the community nurse to come out and do the job, it didn't seem to me to be the best use of her time when I could likely do it myself. I decided to try. If it proved too daunting then I'd have to ask for help.

I took the view that if Mum found it uncomfortable, she'd soon let me know. My mother proved to be as good as gold about the whole undignified process. Sometimes she didn't need any help, but more often than not she did.

Bathing was now only done every two weeks, because Mum was finding the hoisting involved tiring and obviously uncomfortable. Washing her hair was the problem, and the only reason I continued with bathing at all. I toyed with the idea of using a specially designed bowl, for people who were bedridden but the rigidity in her body meant Mum wasn't able to lie in the position required to make this work effectively.

We muddled through as best we could. The meagre baths were now supplemented with bed baths, which had the advantage of being able to combine washing with the massage of limbs anointed with creams.

One night during the winter, after eating her tea, we had a power cut. I was en route to the kitchen with a tray full of dishes and for a split second was brought to a halt, disorientated by the sudden blackout. From the bedroom came a plaintive cry.

'Mum! Mum!'

She hadn't spoken any words for months. Her vocabulary had not been extensive, most words having disappeared before she came into my care in 2001. A very quiet "Yes" or "No" was about her limit and even that had disappeared sometime during the last twelve months. I'd been "Mum" up until a short way through her time in Huesneath Moor and then it was gone. I can't, even now, think of that cry in the darkness without welling up.

'It's okay sweetheart, I forgot to put a shilling in the meter,' I said.

I dumped the tray in the kitchen and went back into the bedroom. By then the lights had come back on and the moment had passed.

January 2004 had been a quiet month. My mother spent much more time in bed and slept for a greater part of the day.

As Jodi put it, 'Joan is winding down.'

Mum still had a healthy appetite, but meal times were taking longer and sometimes it was difficult to tell, when she refused to open her mouth, if she'd had enough to eat or was simply too weary to be bothered. I was contemplating this conundrum while I attempted to feed her with a pot of strawberry trifle one evening.

'Tell me if you've had enough,' I said.

I spoke the words into the ether, never expecting a reply. By coincidence or design, my mother's face puckered up in an expression of distaste. I laughed at her appropriate response and gave her a hug.

'I do love you, you know.'

I couldn't remember ever telling Mum that I loved her. The feeling of genuine warmth and affection that I felt for her in that moment were emotions I normally kept well submerged. Bringing them to the surface had taken me by surprise. I beat a hasty retreat to the kitchen to regain control.

***

It was almost three years since my mother had come to live with me and her night routine had remained the same throughout. She was settled to sleep earlier these nights, though she dozed through much of the day.

At around 8pm I'd turn her onto her right side with her back to the door. I'd turn off her music and the fibre optic lamp that threw a rainbow of colours onto the wall and ceiling. It was on loan from Jake's collection of retro gear. Mum was usually asleep by the time I'd cleared away the evidence of the day. I'd pull her door to, not closed, but enough to cut out noise and light to her room. Then I'd slump into her recliner and succumb to exhaustion until the cold woke me.

The central heating went off at 10pm. My mother had an oil filled radiator in her bedroom which kicked in when the heating clicked off. The cold air would tug against my desire to remain unconscious at about 1am. Mum would be changed, given a drink and resettled on her other side. Then I'd collapse into bed. By this time I could complete the whole routine in snooze mode. Once my head collided with my pillow, I was out cold.

This particular night I must have been so exhausted that I didn't wake until nearly 3am. It'd never happened before, but I was tired all the time these days, every action was like wading through sludge. Dazed with weariness, I struggled to stand up, then waited for my brain to catch up with my legs, and stumbled towards Mum's bedroom.

The light from the hallway threw a weak glow into the room, enough to accomplish what I needed to do. There was the lingering smell of vanilla air freshener. The motor for the mattress was noisy again, usually a precursor to it packing up altogether, which would be the third one we'd managed to make redundant.

I walked towards the bed to let down the cot sides that prevented her falling. Before I reached the bed I knew there was something wrong, but my brain couldn't put words to it.

Mum seemed to be turned too far into the pillow, was that it? Or was it the underlying nothingness beneath the hum of the motor. No movement. No sound. My heartbeat escalated, my limbs wouldn't obey me. In a tense, uncoordinated movement I turned and fumbled with the switch, flooding the room with harsh, unforgiving light.

I began to talk to her, as I touched her left shoulder, warm through the T-shirt she was wearing. I walked round to the other side of the bed, talking to her all the time, I told her how sorry I was for coming in late to change her, sorry that I'd fallen asleep, sorry that I'd failed to hear her distress.

We were now face to face, but not really, as her face was turned into the pillow. I put my arms underneath her, aware of the warmth and moisture of her body, and in a perfected move, I turned my mother to face the ceiling.

Her eyes weren't quite shut, there were white slits showing beneath her eyelids. The side of her face that had rested in the pillow was purple and the right side of her nose was squashed in, restricting her airway.

I lowered the bed and lay next to my mother on the mattress that was still breathing useless air. I embraced her body and hugged her towards me. I couldn't stop saying sorry. Over and over I intoned this word. Why? What was I sorry for? My mother's life had no quality, her mind had gone, body and brain disconnected, non functioning, obsolete. No, I knew why this sense of remorse was so strong. I was full of self-doubt. When I'd put Mum to bed, I must have failed to position her correctly. How else could she have ended up with her face pushed into the pillow?

There were people to contact. I didn't use the phone in her bedroom, as if I was reluctant for Mum to overhear this conversation. I went into the lounge where, twenty minutes earlier, I'd been oblivious to the events unfolding in the adjoining room. I rang the on-call doctor.

'I'm ringing to report the death of my mother. I live with her as her carer, and I think I've killed her.'

It seemed that I'd scarcely put the receiver down when the doctor arrived. He made his official pronouncement of the obvious and attempted to calm me down. He explained that it was very unlikely that anything I'd done or hadn't done would have made any difference to the outcome. Then the words I knew were coming, but didn't want to hear.

'Because your mother hasn't seen a doctor for some time, she'll have to be moved to the mortuary for a postmortem examination. Under the circumstances, the police will need to be in attendance until the undertakers arrive. Meanwhile, you can't go back into the bedroom.'

'But she must be soaking,' I said. 'I'd gone in to change her. Can't I just wash my mother and put a nightdress on her?'

I was wailing my distress, though I already knew the answer, but the thought of her leaving here, in a grotty old T-shirt soaked in body fluids, compounded my grief. It made no logical sense, obviously any titivating I did here would be undone on the mortuary slab. I was running on raw emotion and fear that I'd been responsible for her death.

***

When the doctor left, I rang Bob and rang and rang. I couldn't rouse him. Eventually, after repeatedly allowing the phone to ring into the answer machine, Bob answered, his voice thick with sleep. I told him what had happened. Did I need him to come over? Only he'd been out celebrating his birthday and was well over the drink drive limit. I said no, but meant yes. In less than half an hour he was at the door, the police arrived not long afterwards.

The two policemen sat at the table in the lounge, while Bob remained out of breathing range lest they detected his alcohol-laden breath. Nice guys, who were slightly ill at ease with this particular assignment. In their minds, it was merely protocol. They didn't guess that they were making polite conversation with a murderer. They had to wait until the coroner's appointed undertakers had removed Mum's body. They were happy to drink tea and eat biscuits until then.

The undertakers arrived. I left Bob to deal with them. I saw the draped chest on wheels, containing my mother in her grotty old T-shirt, go past the glazed lounge door. That was more than enough for me.

The police left, but I was high on caffeine and fear, too keyed up for bed. Bob and I stayed put, reminiscing and planning the future, the funeral arrangements and beyond. Bob went home before the work traffic got moving, aware that he'd still be over the limit. I continued to sit, unwilling to think or motivate myself to move. It was over. I felt empty, drained of all emotion.

***

I decided to ring Jodi. She was due in that morning and I didn't want her to have a wasted journey. Of course, she came in anyway, shaky and tearful. We sat and drank coffee, but I was on edge and would remain so until I'd heard from the coroner. I'd been told not to expect a result that day, but it would be impossible to settle to anything until I knew one way or the other.

Jodi persuaded me to help her dismantle the mattress, wash and pack it, ready for collection by the local Health Authority. I'd already agreed with Bob that we'd donate the bed to the hospital, so Jodi and I deep cleaned it and cleared away the paraphernalia of care giving from my mother's bedroom.

Physically, we kept busy, but my mind was on the telephone, willing it to ring. Jodi went home. I'd agreed with Bob that we'd give her an extra month's pay, in lieu of notice, as soon as we could release funds. All Mum's assets would be frozen until we could produce certified copies of the death certificates and the will.

Friends drifted in and out throughout the day, as the bush telegraph kicked into action. Bob came back, as he'd promised he would. Late in the afternoon, I received a phone call from the coroner's office. The woman's efficient voice was tempered with compassion.

'I understand you're anxious to know the cause of death,' she said. 'It was coronary artery atheroma with a secondary cause, which was Alzheimer's disease.'

'My mother didn't suffocate then?' I asked.

'I know you were afraid that may have happened, that's why I'm ringing you. Let me explain. When your mother died, her body lost all resistance and became a dead weight and that pulled her over into the pillow, nothing sinister. I hope that puts your mind at rest.'

It did. I was elated. An inappropriate reaction given the circumstances. I came off the phone and actually did the "Yes!" thing, punching the air. Friends looked at me somewhat perplexed, I hadn't told them the details.

In the same week that Mum died, my decree absolute came through.

Time to move on.

Mum
Born 26th February, 1920 – Died 3rd February, 2004.

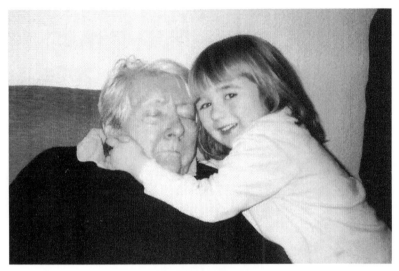

Mum and Sharnie

If you enjoyed this book, please consider leaving a review.
Thank you!

The author can be contacted at jillstoking@gmail.com

Website
http://joansdescent.weebly.com